D0296119

Dear Michael, Love Dad

Dear Michael, Love Dad

IAIN MAITLAND

HODDER &
STOUGHTON

First published in Great Britain in 2016
By Hodder & Stoughton
An Hachette UK company

1

Copyright © Hug Me Limited 2016

The right of Iain Maitland to be identified as the Author of the Work has been asserted by him in accordance with the Copyright, Designs and Patents Act 1988.

All rights reserved. No part of this publication may be reproduced, stored in a retrieval system, or transmitted, in any form or by any means without the prior written permission of the publisher, nor be otherwise circulated in any form of binding or cover other than that in which it is published and without a similar condition being imposed on the subsequent purchaser.

A CIP catalogue record for this title is available from the British Library

Hardback ISBN 978 1 473 63816 7
Trade paperback ISBN 978 1 473 63817 4
Ebook ISBN 978 1 473 63818 1

Typeset in Electra LT by Hewer Text UK Ltd, Edinburgh
Printed and bound by Clays Ltd, St Ives plc

Hodder & Stoughton policy is to use papers that are natural, renewable and recyclable products and made from wood grown in sustainable forests. The logging and manufacturing processes are expected to conform to the environmental regulations of the country of origin.

Hodder & Stoughton Ltd
Carmelite House
50 Victoria Embankment
London EC4Y 0DZ

www.hodder.co.uk

PREFACE

What This Book Is – and Most Definitely Isn't

This is the story of a father and son, Iain and Michael Maitland, covering the years when Michael went to university, his descent through mental illness into hospital and, finally, the Priory. Told through a mix of letters, emails and a commentary, it describes an ordinary, loving family almost torn apart.

This is not a misery memoir. We don't want sympathy or pity.

This is not a self-help book for anyone with mental health issues. We do not have the answers.

This is not a how-to book for parents of children with depression or anorexia. We cannot tell anybody what to do.

This book does not contain any words of wisdom, common-sense advice or guidance for anyone. It is written by an idiot.

This is a story about love – irritated and annoyed, sometimes tender and thoughtful, occasionally bemused and exasperated, and most often long-suffering, but always about love. The book is funny and angry, caustic at times, but it is warm-hearted and open, and shines a light on a close and caring family with love at its heart.

It's about love, remember.
That's all you need to know.

Iain Maitland
Suffolk, July 2016

PS There are a few words of wisdom – not from me, obviously, but from Michael – at the end of the book.

*For Tracey, Michael, Sophie, Adam
and those we've loved and lost.*

ACKNOWLEDGEMENTS

I must thank Tracey, Michael, Sophie, Adam and Niamh for letting me tell our story as I saw it with only a few minor tweaks.

I would like to thank my agent, Clare, who saw this book for what it is: a love story. We met for breakfast and you said you'd start pitching the book and keep going until there were no publishers left. I couldn't have asked for more. The next morning . . .

Hannah, your response took my breath away. I am grateful for your advice and guidance, and for steering me where I needed to go. I couldn't have wished for a better editor.

Thanks, too, to all the team at Hodder – Liz, Louise *et al* – for your work on this book. Sarah, I love your cover! Thank you, Hazel, for your copyediting.

I thank Dr Peter Webster at The Priory Hospital Chelmsford for giving me permission to reproduce his emails to me.

I would also like to thank Becky Bagnall: you showed enthusiasm and pointed me in the right direction when I'd given up and thrown it away.

Jayne Davey, at Suffolk User Forum: you offered help and kindness, and reached out at the darkest time; thank you.

Suzanne Hope, thank you for the work you do with Michael.

Special thanks to Michael. I could not have written this book without his blessing, which he gave with enthusiasm. He also provided notes from his diary on page 337 and his thoughts on the book on page 343.

THE BEGINNING

I'd like to start at the beginning, the day that Michael was born. I should say Michael was always a handsome young man. But I didn't always think so. I remember the moment of his birth. As he was lifted up towards us by the midwife, I looked at that intense, screwed-up face, purple and smeared with blood, and whispered to my wife, Tracey, 'He's a bit ugly, isn't he?' I forget, for the moment, her exact words of reply.

Michael, so far as I understood, had a contented childhood. We lived, in succession, in nice homes close to the sea in Suffolk. He went to good schools. He had friends. He was followed, four years later, by a sister, Sophie, and a brother, Adam, seven years after that. We had days out, weekend trips and regular holidays. Tracey and I have had a long and happy marriage. We've been together since schooldays, when we were fifteen and eighteen respectively.

Michael left home to start his degree in Norwich, Norfolk, in 2007. He was joined by a live-in girlfriend, Niamh. All seemed well for a while. Eventually, and it took us a long, long time to notice, let alone realise what was going on, we saw a change in his appearance and demeanour. It was clear he was not eating properly and that he was getting thinner. As time passed, more serious issues were developing. Anorexia wasn't the half of it.

I struggled to understand and support him during this time. I instructed him. Cajoled him. Humoured him for a long while. At times, too many times and for far too long, I tried to ignore what was happening. At others, such as when he chose not to come to his grandmother's funeral, I raged and threatened to have him sectioned and sent to a mental institution. With hindsight, that might have been for the best but I couldn't bring myself to do it. I got no further than the GP's surgery. I always had a 1960s image of strait-jackets, rubber pipes and force-feeding in my mind.

Gradually, without anything ever really being said, we all seemed to resign ourselves to what we knew deep down would be the inevitable and tragic ending. The call – a text, really – came one day, an evening just after six o'clock, Hallowe'en-time. He had always loved Hallowe'en. By now wraithlike, Michael had succumbed to pneumonia and had been taken into hospital. Our son was about to die.

Michael lived.

But there was worse to come.

The Priory, and a journey into Hell and heartbreak.

But we will come to that, and more, later.

I wrote letters, some emails and notes to Michael during these years. In many ways, they tell of his descent, in free-fall really, a father's ignorance and stupidity, and a once joyous family almost torn apart by tragedy.

Let me show you some of these with a behind-the-scenes commentary. They tell you our story, from a happy beginning through those sad and terrible times as Michael went to the edge of grief and sanity, to the proverbial Hell.

I have tried to tell Michael's story as truthfully as I can. In particular, I have not wanted to put harrowing information – tubes, drips, needles – into the public domain. I may be an unreliable narrator. But my biased and arm's length perception of what happened will not be the same as Michael's reality and truth (which he shares with us towards the end of the book).

We stand now, united again as a family, somewhere in a dark tunnel. We hold hands. We whistle loudly. We have torches. Somewhere, not so very far away, we can see the light. Sometimes it seems close to us. At others it seems a long way off. We will walk into that light together. It will not be tomorrow, or next week, but I'm sure it will happen one day. I hope it will be soon. It will be the best day of our lives.

THE MAIN CAST

Michael: Michael Maitland

'You should be in some sort of institution. You clearly do not function in any way, shape or form. You do not work . . . You seem to have no thought for anyone around you.'

Dad: Iain Maitland

'I had not realised, until I saw the holiday photos, that I now have a bald patch to add to all my other woes . . . I then mentioned it in passing, very casually, and your mother and Adam both said in unison . . . "We know, we didn't like to mention it." I don't know where I go from here – billiard-ball bald, I imagine. It is all too much at times.'

(Dear) Mother: Tracey Maitland

'I know, from hard-won experience, that she thinks she has long arms, a short waist and 'average' length legs and that she does not like the way she walks. This, when written down, suggests more than a passing resemblance to an orangutan but I think you'll agree this is a little harsh.'

Sophie: Michael's younger sister

'Sophie has taken to wearing bright red lipstick inexpertly applied. She reminds me and Adam of the Joker in *Batman*. We have not said anything – even in a seemingly cheerful mood, she can turn very quickly.'

Adam: Michael's younger brother

'I've been trying to drill it into him that he's not stupid but that he has dyscalculia. He's been trying to use that as an excuse with the teachers to get out of anything he doesn't want to do: games, cross-country running, work.'

Bernard: the family Jack Russell

'Bernard needs walking twice a day. I do seven thirty and about six in the evening. If you go much beyond that, he will sit in front of you and stare until you give in. Don't take him on. I've tried. He wins.'

THE SUPPORTING CAST

Niamh: Michael's girlfriend

Granny: Michael's grandmother, Iain's mother

Alf: Granny's former boyfriend

Grandad Terry: Granny's second husband

Ray and Peter: Grandad Terry's sons

Nan: Granny's mother

Grandpa: Granny's father

Roger: Granny's brother

Auntie Queenie: Nan's sister and suspected vampire

Grandma: Michael's maternal grandmother, Tracey's mother

Lee: Sophie's first boyfriend

Henry Beaumont III: Sophie's second boyfriend

Paul: Sophie's third boyfriend

Kathy and Mark Robertson: former friends of the family

Megan Robertson: daughter of Kathy and Mark Robertson

(Little) George: Megan's younger brother

Most of the supporting cast have had their names and, where appropriate, some identifying facts changed to protect their privacy. These facts are largely irrelevant to the essence and flow of the story.

2007

At the start of 2007, I'd been a freelance writer for some twenty years, and spent most of my time writing a range of wealth, health and happiness articles for various magazines and newsletters no one has ever heard of, let alone read. That, and looking out to sea from my bedroom window, watching the boats go by.

Tracey, having raised the children – Michael was now nineteen, Sophie fifteen and Adam eight – was working full-time as a teaching assistant at a local primary school. She'd previously worked part-time for a photographic studio, and with children who had Down's Syndrome or other issues.

Michael was completing a pre-degree art course at the local college in Ipswich. Sophie was doing her GCSEs, with her results due the following summer. She was head girl at her school and was expecting to get straight As in everything. Adam was at prep school, studying something, no one quite knew what, not even his teachers.

We holidayed as a family in Orlando, Florida, for three weeks at Easter, with another family, the Robertsons. We thought, having been away at Easter and in the summer for around twenty years, this might be our last family holiday together. It did not, for one reason or another, go well with the Robertsons – we will draw a discreet veil over these matters – and our friendship ended.

The rest of the year was happy enough – we went out for days as a family, trips to football matches and theatres in London (plus hours and hours at the Tower of London, following my dear wife who had to read every single sign and piece of paper on offer). Michael played football some weekday evenings and on Sundays. He did karate once a week and had some part-time work in a local restaurant. Happy days – which we took for granted.

And so we come to the autumn of 2007, seemingly a contented family with much to look forward to. Michael was the first of our children to leave home and, as he had a talent for drawing, we envisaged him doing his degree and going on to have a successful career as an illustrator. Ready for take-off, he was going just one way – upwards. We wanted our children to fly free, knowing that we were there if they needed us. That was what we expected to happen and it's where we begin our story.

30 September 2007

Dear Michael,

Moving your whatnots et al into the flat has put paid to any improvement in my back. I think the advantages of being on the third floor (nice views of the city) may be outweighed by the disadvantages of trying to heave a wardrobe, a bed and what have you up and around what must be the narrowest staircases known to man. Still, at least it's done now.

Your mother is already worrying how you will cope and is at work on reams of notes on all sorts of matters from how to tell if meat has gone off to washing whites. Smell it and wear black (less washing) is my advice. No doubt you will ask us as you usually do before anything troubles you unduly. Please do try to master the can opener and other basics before calling. You know how your mother worries. I really don't want to be doing round-trips at night to unblock sinks and change fuses. Refer to that AA Handy DIY book first. It may be old but not much has changed and it has stood me in good stead for the past twenty-five years.

Hopefully, that wodge of cash will see you through until your student money comes in. I cannot imagine what you will need it for as you seem to have bagged all of our weekly shop. Try not to fritter money away. Save a little each week. It soon adds up. I am sure you will find there are many distractions when you start college, and lots of rogues and ne'er-do-wells will try to part you from your limited resources. As a rule of thumb, people – students and lecturers these days – with tattoos and piercings are best avoided. We're talking ex-prisoners and sailors mostly. Keep away from anyone with dilated pupils too. They're a tell-tale sign.

I have looked up the Norwich School of Art and Colouring In on the internet and it seems to offer the wide range of arts and crafts you enjoy doing. I do hope you will use your time wisely and come out the other end if not self-supporting at least with a job of some kind. I know nobody really wants to do a job unless they enjoy it but sometimes you simply have to try.

We will come up and see you on your birthday and take you out for the usual slap-up meal. Do have a mooch around and see if you can find somewhere close by that doesn't just have pizzas and burgers on the menu. Your mother will call you to make the arrangements. Adam and Sophie send their love and are looking forward to the meal.

Love

Dad

x

PS I will write again, probably on Sundays when I have a few quiet moments to myself. By the by, I enclose a sponsorship form for Adam. Fill it in and send it back, will you? No doubt I will end up paying for every Maitland on the list. I can but hope.

I began writing letters in the mid-1970s. They became so profuse that, by the end of the decade, it was widely rumoured within the family that Great Aunt Queenie, a regular recipient of five- and six-page thank-you letters after birthdays and Christmases, had begged my grandmother to stop me sending them. I did not, although I did reduce the number of pages (and filled one side only, no longer both).

It all started when Nan and Grandpa moved away from London to the Sussex coast in the 1970s. I used to see them every weekend until then but after that, with my parents divorced (messily, with lots of anger and bitterness) and ghastly new spouses on the scene, I only saw them in the school holidays when I stayed with them.

Without a phone in my mother's home until about 1978 – we did have running water and an inside toilet, thankfully – I wrote to Nan most Sundays with my news and now I wanted to do the same with Michael when he went to university.

Everything I wrote was really for my own pleasure and amusement. Having spent so many years writing about the benefits of putting Vaseline up your nose and spreading pig manure on your roof extension, the letters were an escape for me. Michael never wrote, being of the email and texting generation, but would do drawings for us from time to time, plus homemade birthday and Christmas cards. We all kept everything.

We thought this would be a time of great excitement and joy for Michael. His whole life lay ahead and he could do just about anything he wanted with his artistic talent. Truth be told, we really had no idea what he was like as a human being. We assumed he was relaxed and confident – he certainly looked it, like a young Greek god. What a time he was going to have.

3 October 2007

Michael,

A mid-week missive of some importance! Your grandmother [Granny] has sent you a birthday card and (I am told) a cheque for a 'substantial sum' to help you to settle into your 'university education' (Granny's words not mine). It has come here and I send it on to you unopened as your new address has not yet done the rounds of family and friends who might give you money.

I am tempted to open the card to see what the 'substantial sum' is. If it were your other grandmother [Grandma], I think we would be talking £50 tops. We have taken bets here – Sophie says £200, your mother comes in at £500 and I fear it may well reach four figures. (Adam suggested £1 million but we can discount that for sure.)

Do give your grandmother a call when you can please; 6 p.m., mid-week, ask vaguely what she's been doing in the garden and if she has been to Worthing lately. Try to make that last question sound as if you are interested in what she is doing rather than implying there is something you want her to get for you next time she is in Worthing.

Do try not to spend the money all at once.

Love

Dad

x

Money is a regular theme from the outset. As mentioned, when Michael was doing A levels, he had held down a part-time job washing dishes in a local restaurant. He was, give or take, self-sufficient. (Hurrah! The dream surely of every long-suffering parent with children in their teens, twenties, thirties, forties . . .)

We had urged him to take up offers to become a waiter – more money, more tips – but he chose to stay in the kitchen. Looking back – and it's easy to see it now – we recognise that this might have had something to do with a lack of confidence on Michael's part.

Once he had gone to Norwich, Michael soon gave up doing any work other than what he had to do for his course. The football, karate and other activities stopped too. The friends drifted away. We supported him financially while he was there – we saw this as our way of helping him get the best degree he could.

As for the rest of it, we left him to 'sort himself out'. Perhaps we shouldn't have done: maybe a more hands-on approach would have been better. But we'd been close and active parents when he and our other children were small, ferrying them about, arranging get-togethers with friends, fussing over them, checking all was well, as so many parents do these days. We wanted to let them be themselves as they grew up, making their own decisions and choices, right or wrong. We wanted to take a background role, there if needed, but not interfering. In short, we stood well back.

1 November 2007

Dear Michael,

We had a steady and surprisingly long queue of assorted mother hens and small children last night mixed in with the usual groups of shaven-headed youths, all bristling with aggression. I resorted to handing out mini Mars Bars to placate them. Judging by the nods and grunts – not one of them makes eye contact or articulates a single word known to mankind – I was successful. Plate cleaned by seven o'clock and we resorted to the bottom of drawers and backs of cupboards for the stragglers. The last trick-or-treater – a tall thin beanpole of a teenager riddled with acne, poor boy – had to make do with a handful of After Eights. The look on his face was priceless.

I am working hard – one of us has to – and have an article being published in the national press next week (I think:

8

they are never too specific). I will save it for you so you can feign interest in due course. It's some nonsense on buying a second hand car at auction, which reminds me to tell you to check your oil and water and tyres at least once a week. It only takes a minute and may well save you a breakdown. When your mother and I were younger and didn't have two pennies to rub together, I had to drive to Oxford to see a publisher. Oil was something of a luxury in those days and the engine duly 'threw a con rod' (as per AA man's assessment). Layman's terms? One buggered-up engine. Result? No car for months. Think about it.

I have been perusing the photographs of the Orlando holiday and notice that, in the photo by that *Jaws* shark at Universal, you looked decidedly sleek. I know the Maitlands are prone to being big-boned and everyone looks thin next to me. Your dear mother, of course, is not fat at all but is undeniably short, which can create an unfortunate effect at times. Looking at the other pictures, you do look as though you have wandered in from another family's photographs. What do you weigh at the moment?

Love

Dad

xx

PS I weigh 110 kilos according to our bathroom scales. Northwards of 15 stones I believe. 110 sounds better and lighter than I actually feel to be honest.

Weight – another theme – rears its head early in our story. We'll come to my weight issues soon enough: I've been asked to step off rides at theme parks – even American ones – and move seats in aeroplanes when, I assume, they had a shortage of ballast for that particular flight.

As for Michael, his weight issues seemed to start around 2006–7 when he moved from the school he'd been at for most of his boyhood to another, which had an 'arty' sixth form college. We meant well – it was the best school we could find for his artwork and photography and we believed he'd be happy there.

Apparently, though, someone said something nasty to him one day about his appearance and that – one tiny, thoughtless comment – might have been the trigger that set him on his endless downward path. I have the Orlando photo in front of me now, as I write these words, and Michael looks slim, not 'thin' – just 'slim'. Clearly, this was the early stages of it all – not that we had grasped it then.

November 2007

Michael,

A brief note about your dear mother's birthday. Please remember it is the 18th. I do not wish to have to run around at the last minute (again) trying to cover for you. This year it is on a Sunday and I wonder if you might honour us with your presence? I enclose a £20 note to this effect. We will be at the Alex at 1 p.m. Your (surprise, surprise) arrival at 1.10 p.m., with a present in hand, please, would be most welcome.

In terms of a card and a present, please try to get a card that has 'Mum' or similar on it. 'You're Just Like a Mother' (*circa* 2004?) does not qualify as 'similar'. As for a present, please do remember how sensitive your mother is about birthdays. Chocolates (weight), skin things (wrinkles) and small-print books (eyesight) are all no-nos. You have done the face mask 'joke' before and that is still relatively fresh in the memory so kindly avoid that one again.

Anyhow, let us hope we see you on the 18th just after 1 p.m. Please liaise with Sophie and Adam so you do not all buy the same thing – unless you want to club together and get something?

Love,

Your Long-Suffering Father

xx

PS If all else fails, bring flowers, but not 'funeral flowers'. It reminds your mother of Grandpa. And not petrol station ones either. Sainsbury's is okay.

Tracey and I have been fortunate that we always seem to have agreed naturally on how to bring up our children – I recall no cross words or disagreements over the years and everything seemed to fall into place when they were small. We did it all instinctively but it seemed to work well.

I wouldn't say we were delighted to see our children leave home but neither were we distraught at the thought of their departure. Certainly, stories in the papers of 'empty nest syndrome' would make us laugh out loud. We saw Michael leaving, then Sophie and eventually Adam as being the natural scheme of things. (Of course, just when you think you've got the place to yourself at last, they all come back, but that's another story for another time.)

With Michael gone, there was still close and regular contact between everyone. He was only just up the road in Norfolk. Tracey and he would talk on the phone – still the landline for us old people in those days – followed later by the mobile and, occasionally, emails. And there was contact between the three children too, a plethora of text speak and smiley faces, which we thought was 'awsm lol'.

November 2007

Dear Michael,

Thank you for coming down – I was not sure you would turn up but was pleased that you did; your choice of card and present were spot-on. Well done. Your dear mother was delighted and is currently on cloud nine. I will make the most of what might be several days of a benign mood to slip in various pieces of bad news I have been saving up for such a time.

I note that your hair has changed colour again. I am all for an 'artistic' look for an art student but would caution you against excessive bleaching and use of chemicals. You do not know the effects of chemicals on your body. Your scalp is like a sponge and these chemicals may well soak through into your bloodstream and be all round your body before you know it.

Your great-grandfather on the paternal side died of rotten teeth. It got into his bloodstream and did for him at fifty-six. None of the Maitland men live past sixty – never have – so you do not want to be doing anything to hasten matters. Think on it, please.

It is nice to see you making your own cards. It was very imaginative. Could you maybe try selling one or two to generate some extra cash? It's a good time of year to be doing Christmas cards. You could perhaps sell them on eBay. Have a word with Sophie? I believe she has sold various unwanted gifts on it.

Love

Dad

PS Some thoughts for Christmas presents, please? I am loath to give money so don't ask for it. You can have one big present and some small ones or lots of small ones. We are trying to cut back a little this year so do not expect Father Christmas to get you everything on your list. You may, as I do, wish to operate a star system. Five stars means a 'must have', four stars means 'I'd like it a lot', and so on. Do not give everything five stars.

All appeared well at this stage, not that we were conscious that things could be anything but. We all seemed to be happy and, if asked, we would have said that we saw ourselves as a normal family.

It was not that we thought we were better than anyone else – although, let's be frank, there are some rough old sorts you see out and about – but that we were all content and everything was moving along as expected.

We were largely oblivious to Michael's weight now and for some time to come – he was 'slim', remember, not 'thin'. We met up for meals regularly – three family birthdays (out of five) are in October and November and everything seemed as it always had.

Michael's appearance – hair, what he wore – was forever changing and had done for two or three years. We took that as an 'age thing' rather than anything more troubling.

It had irritated us a little in the past – the bleach on the towels, the floor and everywhere else – but it had mostly amused us, not least the day Michael's hair turned orange and I had to dash to a chemist to buy a box of brown hair dye to turn it back (and to face the withering look of the woman behind the counter, who obviously felt that Warm Auburn was the first tell-tale sign of a midlife crisis). We never took it as being anything other than normal, though. Kids, eh?

December 2007

Dear Michael,

We have been playing happy families, all trooping in regularly to see the latest blockbusters on Sundays. We have seen *The Golden Compass*, which was quite good but I fell asleep somewhere in the middle and lost track of the plot.

Adam has taken to perusing past and future film titles on the internet and has been matching them up with various family members. He is *I Am Legend*. Sophie is *Don't Touch the Axe* (can you imagine?). You are matched with a film called *My Kid Could Paint That*.

Niamh lives in a house in darkest Norfolk with a moat around it? I don't doubt that this is a step up for you socially – you'll not be able to take a girl like that to the Wimpy Bar for a Bendy Burger and a Brown Hat. But I urge you to be cautious.

In my experience, these rural families are invariably up to their eyeballs in debt. You may well aspire to taking over as Lord of the Manor but you will invariably end up as Lord Muck. You cannot simply sit back and wait for money to come to you – you have to work at it.

Adam went on a school trip. Text me, I said, when the coach leaves Cambridge Services. I can then finish off the decorating (hall, stairs, landing – cream), get washed and be there for you when you get back to school. Text duly arrives: *Be there in 10 minutes*. Mad panic and on the way to school in paint-smeared clothes at 80 m.p.h. Off the bypass and on the way to school and the next text arrives: *Now at Cambridge Services*. Turned car round at ski slope, repeated process an hour later. My, how we laughed. *I Am Legend*? *Dumb and Dumber* more like.

Love

Dad

x

PS When you visit a house with a moat, check to see if it is full of water and relatively clean. If the moat is overgrown and full of broken bicycle parts and spare tyres, they don't have any money. Think on it.

And so we end the year with Niamh. She moved in with Michael in Norwich in 2007 and quickly became the most important person in his life.

A few years earlier, Tracey had seen a psychic and he'd said that we – Tracey and I – were 'like two swans, who mate for life'. We soon came to see Michael and Niamh in much the same way.

We thought it was good for Michael to be part of a couple. Company for him, we said. And Niamh was arty and confident and outgoing too – so, a perfect match and balance. As we moved into 2008, things were looking good. Life, frankly, was as happy as it had ever been. We had it all.

2008

We had high hopes for Michael as the year began: he was living with Niamh in a flat we'd bought in Norwich and really had everything going for him. We saw him fairly often and all seemed well. His appearance changed regularly but we gave that little or no thought, other than making references to him looking like famous people (mostly wild-eyed serial killers).

As for the rest of us, life continued much as usual – an ordinary life. Tracey loved working with small children, mostly sweet and good-natured, at the local primary school. Sophie was gearing up to achieve the most and highest-graded GCSEs ever known in the UK, along with a mention in *The Guinness Book of Records*, quite possibly the world version. Adam was attempting to put fingers in both ears and both nostrils at the same time and was determined to achieve it.

I was writing articles advising readers on how to be healthy, get rich and be happy although I could only really tick the 'happy' box for myself. For 'happy', you could really say 'blissfully ignorant': the signs were there already, if only we'd looked. We never really noticed. Our family was a cheerful one and nothing bad could ever happen to us.

6 January 2008

Dear Michael,

January – post-Sophie's birthday, of course – is always a
miserable affair. Christmas has been and gone. So too are
the decorations. Everyone has gone back to work and
school – join-the-dots college in your case – and I sit here
on my own, staring out to sea at overcast skies and grey
waters. Business is dead and I have the tax returns to do
and payments to make which I spent on Christmas.

So, I've decided – not mentioned it yet to your dear
mother – we will go back to Orlando again this year. I
think, after last year's fiasco, that we need to go again asap.
Otherwise we will never return and all our memories of
America will for ever be tainted by the holiday from Hell.
We will do three weeks in August in a villa like last year's
but nicer – I have found several near Haines City, the opposite end of the I4 to last year (Clermont).

Would you and Niamh like to come? I'd pay for your
flights and food and Universal tickets – not Disney this
time, which is nice but better for smaller children, really –
and everything else. (D'uh, obviously.) Can you at least
bring some spending money of your own, though, so you're
not hustling me for dollars every five minutes when we are

there? Can Niamh or her folks pay for her flights and maybe the Universal tickets if we take care of 'board and lodgings'? (I can't be doing with separate bills and two dollars of this and a dollar of that for what she's eaten.) I can be arm-twisted a little on all of this as I'd like us to have a nice proper family holiday together but not too much, please.

You know little Olivia, don't you? I imagine we will invite her (if all are agreeable), not least because Sophie has been to St Tropez with her family. I got away with just paying for flights and dropping £100 cash in a wad of folded-up fivers to the father but you can spend that on a round of Cokes in the South of France so I will pick up the tab for Olivia this time.

Did Sophie tell you that Olivia's dad was in a pop group called Modern Romance years ago? They were quite big at the time. I can't remember the whole of their best song but I recall singing the main line, 'best years of our lives', to your mother when we lived the other side of London. As I was unemployed for almost three years, 1982 to 1985, I suspect they weren't.

If you YouTube 'Modern Romance, Top of the Pops' you will find stuff by them. Rob is on keyboards and looks like Princess Diana. You'd not recognise him. See what you think. Morrissey once said something like 'There are worse groups than Modern Romance but can anyone really think of one?' I liked them, though.

He's a nice fellow – he set up and ran, then sold and bought back, some media agency in the City. Whenever our paths cross and we chat, he seems to be doing PR deals with stars like Elton John and Sting whilst I've been writing articles about eating soup with a fork and putting cow pats on your head ('5 Amazing Ways To Cure Baldness Once & For All!'). How the other half lives. When Olivia did the last 'Go to Work with Your Parents' day, I think she was working near Liam Neeson whilst Sophie helped me rod the drains because some fool had been shoving floor wipes down the cloakroom toilet.

At the dentist's – is there an unfilled tooth in my head? – I read a celebrity airhead interview in one of these 'my gerbil ate my boyfriend' magazines. Why does 'being happy' always involve winning the lottery? And why does everyone always have to be happy all the time anyway? I'm not. I'm not sure I'd want to be. It would annoy your mother, having me keep laughing and guffawing to myself all the time.

All for now,

Dad

My mind drifts to what Michael was like as a little boy. There are many happy memories.

The 4 a.m. bottle feed when he was a month old – I'd swear he looked at me, focused, and smiled. A song, Fleetwood Mac's 'Little

Lies', played in the background. In difficult times, I couldn't listen to it. Still can't, really.

Later, when I gave him an evening bath, I'd hold his legs and pull him gently back and forth through the bubbles so the water would wash over his face; he'd laugh and splutter in delight.

A kite in a park in Littlehampton, near my mother's, the first and last time I'd ever got one to fly high in the wind. Michael's hands outstretched, clapping with joy.

Walking through foot-deep snow outside our home, so much snow that I had to lift and carry him at times; snowballs and snowmen with satsumas, twigs and stones for buttons. Freezing cold hands and hot chocolate.

Driving to see *The Sooty Show*, Michael calling out, 'Faster, Daddy, faster,' so we'd see him sooner. Delight when Matthew Corbett made a joke with Tracey – the perils of being on the front row.

A little older, now nicknamed 'Mucker', all of us singing our own version of the 'Rock Me Amadeus' song as we drove for hours up and down the A12, M25 and M23, to visit Michael's granny and my grandpa (Granny's father).

Chasing him round the lounge, me on my backside using my legs as crab-like monster pincers; Michael squealing as I caught him and chopped him up.

Kicking a ball on the green opposite our home. Going up and down in the lift when I worked at Suffolk College. Chips and dollops of ketchup in the canteen afterwards. Films we saw every Wednesday matinée before Michael started school.

The happiest of times, which I'd thought would go on for ever.

27 January 2008

Dear Michael,

First things first – Orlando, here we come. Yours truly has pencilled in the holiday for 10 to 31 August – after last year's hoo-hah, having to run like billy-o to catch the connecting flight, we are flying direct and on a Sunday too (cheaper). I have semi-sorted the villa – i.e. I emailed the owner this week who says it is free – and now just need to crack on and book the flights. Can you talk to Niamh so we can get this all booked up by the end of this week? If you give your dear mother a call, maybe Wednesday, she can tell you more and we can confirm various website addresses and what have you so you can see what's what.

Does Niamh have a passport? I need her full name and date of birth and the passport number and start and end dates of it to book flights. I'd like to fly Virgin if possible; I think their seats are a little larger so I can sit there without having my stomach hanging over the edges.

I am still swimming although I cannot say much is happening weight-wise. I try to do thirty minutes of breast stroke a day, which some dodgy website or other seems to suggest burns up 370 calories; thirty minutes of that compares to seventy-five calories if I walk at 2 m.p.h. (that's plenty), 180 calories if I cycle at 10 m.p.h. (that's not happening) and 300 calories if I run at 6 m.p.h. (let's all laugh).

I can only do breast stroke – with front crawl, I veer to the left (it may have something to do with being left-handed) and, if the pool were not roped into three lanes (old dears, normal people, maniacs), I imagine I would eventually go round in a complete circle. The butterfly is just silly (and quite possibly a physical impossibility for me given the girth).

Your mother is not best pleased with me. A catalogue came through the door for the glorious House of Bath and they had a range of nice-looking boots on the front. Think Adam Ant (eighties fop). A good price too – so I suggested your dear mother might like to buy a pair with my card (Brownie points in the bag for when she spots the recent car damage where I reversed into a post in someone's driveway in Kirton, long story). Bad move – not only did they, I am reliably informed, look like something 'an old lady' might wear but I had not read the small print. Apparently, they have Velcro fittings to help undo and do up the boots. Sounds good to me but your mother is unduly sensitive about her age. I beat a hasty retreat.

Some news of Sophie and Adam. We think Sophie and Lee are getting serious; he seems like a nice boy. Before they got together, he came round and introduced himself and we all shuffled about awkwardly. He does tennis at the club and goes to that school – name escapes me for the moment – up near the hospital. (Not the one where I used to teach part-time and they used to set fire to each other when the adults' backs were turned.) Your mother likes him and has started buying bits and pieces (cheesy pizzas, microwave burgers) for when he comes over. I am not sure we should be too encouraging in case he turns out to be some sort of deviant. Given his attachment to Sophie, it stands to reason he cannot be all there.

We have, for some time, been seeking something nice and encouraging to say to Adam. He tends not to do too well at school and rather than referring to him as 'a useless great lump' (I plead guilty to multiple offences) it's better, according to one of his right-on teachers, to find something he's good at and focus on that. It's taken some time but at last we've found it. He can stand up straight with his right leg facing forward and his left leg facing backwards; so his feet are in opposite directions. I have told him when he is older he will be able to join a freak show. He seemed quite pleased.

All for now – do call your mother on Wednesday evening. No particular time.

Love

Dad

x

Michael was always a gentle and trusting soul. I remember when he was four or five and the two of us were in Woolworths in Ipswich. We were standing at the videos by the front doors. There was a

Pinocchio one – not the Disney version – and if you pressed a red button, a jewel lit up. Exciting stuff (for me, anyway, pressing it repeatedly and, quite possibly, making a honking noise each time).

I turned and Michael had gone. I checked up and down the aisles. No sign. Looked out of the doors, along the street. Nowhere to be seen. I crossed the store, back and forth. Still no sign. By this time, I was starting to panic. I spoke to a girl behind the counter and said I'd lost my little boy but she smiled vacantly back at me as if I'd said I'd lost tuppence.

I wasn't far off panic although I continued walking up and down looking for Michael as nonchalantly as I could. To be honest, I didn't know what to do. In those days, people didn't make a fuss. Since Princess Diana died, everyone has to let everything out. Now they'd be hollering and shouting and threatening to sue everyone in sight. I just stood there, sweating.

Anyhow, happy ending. Michael marched back into the store hand in hand with two other small children and a mum and dad; he'd tagged on to them, followed them out of the store and all the way down the high street. I could barely speak my words of thanks.

3 February 2008

Michael,

How are you? We were thinking of coming up to Norwich on a Sunday in a week or two's time. We could maybe have lunch at one of those places by the Riverside and then see a film? What is coming up, do you know? Have a think, see what's what, talk to Sophie.

Valentine's Day is fast approaching and you will need to give some careful consideration to it as this will be your first with a real woman (as you may have guessed by now, but maybe not – you were fifteen for Father Christmas – that it was your mother sending those cards all through your teenage years).

Here is my hard-earned Valentine's know-how built up over twenty-eight gruelling years.

Don't give a voucher – it is far and away the most practical gift but it scores low on the romance chart.

Ditto cashola.

Clothes – risky unless you know sizes and there is little or no variation in weight (if you go too small, she'll think she's fat, if you go too big, she'll think you think she's fat). And never buy trousers for a woman. Fatal. Your mother thinks she has long legs like Joanna Lumley. They are more like Jimmy Krankie's (short woman dressed as a schoolboy – don't ask).

Perfume – probably the safest bet; you may get away with a small bottle if you say you wanted to get one to fit her handbag. Just.

Make-up – potentially tricky: you have to avoid anything to do with lines, greasy skin and sagging. Avoid spot and blemish treatment. Keep it upbeat and positive. Talk to a sister or a friend before making your choice. Brands seem to be important to women. It's not just 'black mascara'.

Handbags – it's a fact of life that no woman can have enough handbags; get something similar to what she has already. But go for a different colour that's close to something else she's just bought (coat, shoes, ideally). She'll think you're thoughtful. (But keep the receipt just in case.)

Shoes – ditto, can never have enough. But these are an impossible choice. Women are not like men (one black, one brown, one trainers, one flip-flops) – they have colours and materials and all sorts of mysterious heels (wedges, cones, slingshots, etc.). All very puzzling and best avoided. No man ever bought the right shoes for a woman.

Lingerie & Things – see shoes.

DVDs & CDs – no woman wants these as a present (especially if it's a movie or music you like – the 'I thought we could watch/listen to it together' line somehow seems to cause grief every time, I can tell you).

Weight – don't buy anything that might allude to a woman's weight. Belts can be lethal (even if you offer to push an extra hole in with a screwdriver). If she says she wants to lose weight, don't take her at face value and get any Slimfast-type stuff. Don't encourage talk of that kind. Women often think that certain, really odd, parts of their bodies are fat – fingers, calves, etc. Best just ignore the whole shebang.

A side note on weight – 'The Eight Stone Rule'. This one's vital. At some stage, a woman will ask 'How much do you think I weigh?' It can come out of the blue at any moment. Be on your guard at all times. Never blurt out what you think. There is only one answer – eight stone. Few women are below eight stone and most are above so it's a flattering reply. (Obviously, if you've got an eighteen-stoner on your hands, the eight-stone reply is not credible so you will need to scale it up appropriately – 'Eleven or twelve stone?' might do the trick.)

As you'll know, having been with your mother since 1879, I am not a 'ladies' man' but I have learned these Valentine rules over many years and often the hard way. They've stood me in good stead and may do the same for you. Give them some careful consideration.

Also, think about us coming up in a week or two and what you'd like to do. Then get in touch with Sophie to sort it out.

Your Dear Old Dad, x

PS Woman-wise, a meal always goes down well (in addition to, not instead of, I'm afraid). Avoid fast-food places, Pizza Hut, etc. Don't go to anything too clichéd, Italian, guitars, roses and all that. Never have spaghetti. Think Doctor Who's Ood. Not nice.

Women, eh. What's it all about? I have met some. Not that many.

February 2008

Hello Michael,

Mother's Day – you are duly expected to be on duty. I have booked a table for the five of us at the Alex for midday. Come to the house for eleven?

We may then head over to Ipswich later to the cinema to see something that your mother likes – i.e. it doesn't involve people's heads being cut off. Have a look and see what there is. Think *The Notepad*. Have you seen it? Dreadful old tosh but your mother likes it. At the end, the elderly lovers lie down on a bed and die together at exactly the same time. What are the chances of that happening? I think your mother sees us going the same way. I imagine it's possible with a double-barrelled shotgun.

Gormless girl in Next the other day. Your mother has 'lost' her Next card (i.e. it's in another handbag somewhere) and asked me to go in and tell them. So I did. I added we were worried that someone may have found it and run up some purchases with it (I could probably live with that as it would be less than your mother spends). The girl asked if your mother had signed the back of the card. I said she had. The girl then reassured me that this made a fraud unlikely as any thief would have to sign a slip before buying anything so signatures could be compared. Um, pause. 'Could a thief not just copy the signature on the card?' Long silence. Hopeless.

My 'good deed' this week? Yesterday. Goth girl. Ipswich. M&S cashpoint. I was behind her and got an earful of an argument with her boyfriend who clearly had done something he was not supposed to have done. Tattooed his face? Safety-pinned his private parts? She was giving him what-for. Anyway, she was so furious that, having tapped all the buttons, she took her card back and walked off in a huff, leaving her £10 sticking out of the machine. A tricky moment as I took the money out holding it at arm's length so that anyone watching could see I wasn't actually stealing it. Having called after her twice, 'Hello?', 'Excuse me?', I ended up chasing her down the street. Was she grateful? Was she heck. She glared at me and snatched it out of my hand without a single word. I wish I hadn't bothered.

Anyway, back to Mother's Day and some thoughts on a present. Your mother has been going on at me to redo the bathroom – huge job, £1000s, far beyond me. I've agreed to paint and 'freshen it up'. Can you knock up a painting? A sea view, duck egg blues? It will go above the toilet. Make it as normal as you can. No Martian landscapes or aliens with distended organs, please.

See you at 11. I will slip you a wodgie for your petrol or train money.

Love

Dad

You could, with the benefit of hindsight, clearly see the man inside the boy.

Michael was always a self-contained, happy-in-himself child, and he loved and had a real eye for drawing. I recall, when he was five, his first teacher, the unfortunately named Mrs Grimm, coming out while I was waiting to pick him up from school and saying how he was very good at drawing and 'already draws like a teenager'.

Inevitably, I came straight back with some feeble joke, asking if he had been found drawing on toilet walls again. Silence. Awkward backtracking. Embarrassing conversation to follow. It turned out that he could draw pretty much any *Simpsons* character you named, both spitting image and to scale. It was as if he had traced them (he hadn't). Remarkable, really, not least because no one on either side of the family was remotely artistic.

As I write, I have a drawing on my wall that Michael did for me a year or two ago. It's of all the Doctor Whos, a host of companions and most of the main baddies, including Daleks. It's staggeringly good. To me, who can barely draw a stick insect, it is a wonderful picture.

9 March 2008

Dear Michael,

What is it with workmen these days (or is it 'work people' to be PC)? After months of your mother nagging about pigeon-grey, encrusted windows, I found a window cleaner. I should have been suspicious from the start, given that it all started with a card through the door and the speed with which he visited (same day). He did the windows on the spot – £30.

£30! How long was he here for that princely sum? Three hours? Two hours? Surely not one hour? No – twenty minutes. Don't waste your time on qualifications and degrees. All that stuff they tell you at school about working hard and getting on and earning 20 per cent more than the average person if you get a degree – all utter rot. Be a window cleaner, make £90 an hour – £720 for an eight-hour day and more than £150,000 a year.

What's more, he wanted another £25 to do the roof – I said no, leave it covered in bird muck and damn your mother. Bottom line? He is not allowed to go up ladders because of 'health and safety issues'. He stands on the ground and uses some sort of hose thing (the ledges are still a murky grey). To reach the upper windows, he had to go halfway up the ladder – why have one if you're not supposed to use it? – and I had to stand on the bottom rung to steady it. Honestly, I would have shaken him off if it weren't for the fact I'd let the house insurance lapse (last quote was ridiculous).

We've also got a handyman – Steve – after I cracked under your mother's constant pressure all winter. The 'to do' list on the fridge reached epic proportions (five pages).

What I want from a handyman is this. I give him a job (new lock, new taps). He comes in, does the job without bothering me. He goes. I pay him. Simple? Not quite. He must be the most boring and is certainly the slowest handyman that ever walked this earth.

He's just put up two alarms. Thirty minutes, he says, tops, for the two. All the electricity has to go off ('health and safety' again) despite the fact that the alarms are on their own circuit and he can just flick a switch under the kitchen cupboards. Okay, I reply, 'I'm working on my computer so if you turn off the electricity now, I will stop and have my lunch.'

'I'll stop and have lunch now too,' he says.

I made the fatal mistake, when he first came round, of being friendly. I think he now wants to be best friends and go to the pub and talk crankshafts.

So, I explain, as patiently as I can, that if we stop for lunch at the same time, I will then have to wait another thirty minutes after that whilst he does the alarms. Anyway, two and a quarter hours later – 135 fat and freaking minutes – the job is done. I sat there in the lounge listening to him huffing and puffing and the running commentary on what he was doing and why and how it was so much harder than it should have been (my fault somehow). 'Iain (Note: never Mr Maitland), who did the plastering?' . . . 'Iain, the fixings are in the wrong place' . . . 'Iain, I can show you the fixings if you like' . . . 'Iain, can you read the instructions?' On and on it went, an endless blur of blunder and cack-handedness. I was pretty much shaking with frustration by the end of it.

I say he's the slowest handyman ever but he's certainly the fastest at getting paid. None of this end-of-the-month stuff with him. He texts me the next morning – 7.30 a.m. – and gives me the price, £160, and can I 'do the usual', i.e. leave the cheque under the front doormat. He's there before 9 a.m. picking it up. I'd ignore his text but he'd only knock and spend the next half-hour telling me what he's going to do that day and where and why. We've still three big jobs to go and I cannot face much more of it.

Love

Dad

Was I an awful father? When Michael was in the early days of school, Mrs Grimm went round the class and asked everyone what their fathers did (I guess it was coming up to Father's Day).

Some worked in London, others did a range of jobs across the financial, banking and legal sectors. Most of them wore suits and ties and did something 'important'. My dad, Michael said, 'sits in his bedroom all day and never comes out', making me sound as though I were some sort of manic depressive or perhaps making bombs to overthrow the government of the day.

As an aside, I suspect these days it would be politically incorrect to talk at school of fathers and Father's Day. A few years later, when Sophie was at a pre-school playgroup, there was absolute uproar when the children were encouraged to make a tissue-paper flower for their fathers. Naturally, some children had fathers at home while others had fathers who had left, were in prison, on the run or whatever. One or two of the single mothers came close to blows with the playgroup organiser. I never got my tissue-paper flower.

Was Michael's decline and fall all my fault? I always felt I was a good father. Each day I woke Michael and we watched TV – *Doctor Who* episodes mostly – over breakfast. I took him to school and collected him. We spent time together in the evenings, football in the garden, larking about and so on. When it came to practical stuff, I ticked all the boxes.

But did I ever hug him? A little when he was small. Did I tell him I loved him? Probably not – I don't recall it anyway. Did I encourage him and make him feel good about himself? Not really. I used to tease and joke with him – banter to me, maybe not so for Michael. Perhaps every thoughtless jokey comment was a blow to his morale. He always seemed to take everything in good spirits but maybe I just assumed that was so. He never really answered back or joined in with the banter, even as he got older. Looking back now on Michael's childhood, I search over and over for clues.

March 2008

Dear Michael,

It's all go here, I can tell you. We – me, Adam and your dear mother – have decided to go up to Nottingham for a couple of days over Easter. They have some sort of exhibition for the *Robin Hood* TV show at the castle and I thought it was about time we went there again as we've not been since we stayed with (Great) Auntie Queenie when you were small. 1988?

Auntie Queenie was the one who died and came back to life when you were about ten. It was all a terrible mix-up. Granny rang one evening and told me that AQ had had a stroke and was in hospital on life support. The next morning, the phone rang at about 7.45 a.m. as I was leaving to take you to school so we left it. Assuming Auntie Queenie was stone cold dead, I sat you both down and sensitively broke the news to you as gently as I could. You asked if we could stop at the Spar for some Nik Naks. As it happened, when I spoke to Granny that night, she said she'd rung to say AQ was feeling a little better. Sophie asked if she had come back as a vampire.

Sophie – who will be staying here to keep an eye on the dog – has now decided that, as she will get eleven or twelve A grade GCSEs (naturally), she will do her A levels at Ipswich School. I had hoped that, after Amberfield, we could switch her into the state system so we could hack a little off the overdraft but we made the rash promise that she could go to any sixth form she wanted. Serves me right. That's what comes from bigging yourself up. We showed her round 'good' local state schools in Ipswich and Woodbridge, plus the two private ones. She went for the most expensive, inevitably.

They have offered her a scholarship. When you hear the word 'scholarship', you tend to think 'free' – at least I did anyway. I was floating on air for two days, as pleased as Punch, until the offer letter arrived. A scholarship is not a freebie: it's something like 20 per cent off the bills. What's worse, it's actually a 'half' scholarship as her and some other smart Alec were deemed equally worthy so they split it in two. I know I should be pleased and proud of the big dollop but all I see is a final demand or else. You have to write a lot of 'How to Cure Hay Fever with a Tub of Vaseline' articles to pay for that.

Still at least it means that Sophie and Adam will be in the same school again. We have had to be leaving at 7.40 in the morning to drop Adam at Ipswich at 8.15 (the earliest he can be dropped off) and to get Sophie back to Amberfield at 8.40 (the latest she can be dropped off). By the time I get home at gone 9 for a swim, I'm exhausted already. It's like driving from London to Brighton every morning before work.

News of your dear mother. The Robertson woman texted her asking if she and Adam would like to join her and Little George at a church morning-service thing. Your mother sent me ahead to drop Adam off whilst she 'got ready' (the Queen is quicker getting ready for the State Opening of Parliament). I had a stilted conversation with Mrs Robertson, which lasted about three minutes. I then left as quickly as I could. Your mother went along for the last twenty minutes of whatever it was and came back and wouldn't speak of it. Whatever happened was grim. Hopefully, that's the end of it.

So, that's what's happening here. We hope you are well and that Niamh is too.

Love

Dad

x

PS There is some talk of Adam doing the violin despite a complete absence of musical interest or ability. They might as well try to get a pig to tap-dance. We are trying to sound vaguely encouraging without actually suggesting he does it. Hopefully, the whole idea will just die a natural death.

It may be that, had I encouraged Michael more through his child-hood, he would have had a better perception of himself. I guess that referring to him as 'a mighty brain' and similar on a regular basis and doing impressions of him walking gingerly after a foot-ball injury do not fall into the category of good parental encouragement.

Thinking about things, one incident from Michael's early years rings some alarm bells, albeit twenty odd years too late. (Skip this next bit if you're eating breakfast, lunch or dinner – or even shovelling down a snack.) When he was four or five, small and sweet, we noticed he had a large hard lump in his stomach. We went to the surgery and 'Dr Tom' – a painfully right-on GP who used the word 'penis' in front of Michael (blank look) when we'd been referring to it as his 'winkie' – said it was, spelling out the letters and number, 'S-H-1-T'. (More blank looks, this time from us.)

It turned out Michael had developed a not uncommon childhood phobia about the toilet and had simply stopped going so that everything had – shall we say? – backed up. We were given some sort of liquid, a variation on castor oil, I guess, and were told to be prepared. At 3 a.m. the next night, there was an explosion from the bathroom that rocked the whole house. (We will leave that story there and you can, as appropriate, return to your food.) That episode shows me that Michael, even at that young age, had the most terrific levels of willpower and determination – imagine holding on until you exploded. It doesn't bear thinking about.

April 2008

Dear Michael,

God almighty, my life is a nightmare right now. I'm talking the School Prom. Here's what happened.

As the head girl's father, I am apparently responsible for arranging the end-of-year prom for all the fifth form girls (or whatever Looney Tunes term is used for it these days). Quite why that's become a tradition, I will never know. What a fat, middle-aged man knows about school proms can be written on the back of a stamp. I wouldn't mind so much but no one told me about it until I got an irate call from some woman at the place it's being held, demanding to know numbers and menus and how many teachers would be in attendance; 'health and safety' (groan).

First I'd heard of anything. It seems that one of the girls had decided, with her parents, to arrange everything. (Fair enough, I'd have gone along with that had I known.) They'd picked a lovely venue and were making all the arrangements and then, I'm not sure what happened or why, they walked away from it all, kindly leaving the venue with my name and number. Cue angry phone call.

So I blabbered through the conversation not knowing what the hell it was about and promising to call back the next day when I was 'up to speed' (i.e. when I'd passed it over to your mother). As the conversation ended, the wretched woman pressed a button and clearly thought the call had been disconnected and she made some derogatory remark about people like me (whatever people like me are like: harassed and cheesed off, I imagine). Inevitably, I could not let that lie so I called her straight back and advised her to make sure the phone was cut off before slagging off clients. She said she hadn't said anything, then that it was not about me, and then that someone else had said it (presumably a ventriloquist who could throw their voice across the room and down the receiver). All in all, not a good start to the process.

It gets worse. The minimum number of attendees is 80 and a non-refundable deposit of £500 has been paid. As there are only 35 girls in the whole of the fifth form, we've somehow got to find another 55 people to attend. Parents, boyfriends, locals, passers-by? Prisoners on the run from Hollesley Bay? If we withdraw, I'll be responsible for refunding the £500 to the school.

There's more. My back-of-a-fag packet calculations suggest we are going to need to charge close to £40 a ticket. That's going to cause uproar, I can tell you. I know there's a perception that private school parents are laid-back and polite – generous too. Not when it comes to money and putting their hands in their pockets, they're not. They're like a pack of starving mongrels. They all want something for nothing and some other poor sucker – me – to do all the work. I will have to prepare a breakdown of how the figures add up in readiness for the inevitable onslaught of abuse.

Of course, the final indignity is that we have to smile and laugh and make out it's all great fun. I suspect when they're sitting next to their teachers, drinking one glass of cola each (no alcohol for under 18s, extra drinks £2.99 each), and I've murdered the girl's father for dropping me in it, they may change their mind. (Then again, they all loved it when I shouted at Colin Nixon for booing Sophie when she was playing his daughter at the tennis club so maybe they'd cheer on a good throttling.) I will update you. No doubt it will get worse.

Love

Your Long-Suffering Father

x

PS And how are you? Sophie tells me you are sculpting this term. Sculpting what? Adam has suggested you sculpt – is that the right word? – my head. You'll need a lot of plaster. Adam measured my head the other night as I want to buy a Panama hat online for the holiday (Marks & Sparks only goes up to XL size). He said my head was 66 inches so I am currently known as the man with the five-foot head. The reality, of course, is that it is 66 centimetres. Still a whopper, though. XXL, I believe. And more besides. It's a wonder I can walk upright.

When Michael was young, he went to three different schools in three years. The first closed after his second year there; not enough pupils. The next would only take boys up to the age of seven. He then went to another school further away in Ipswich. I wonder now whether that might have shaken his confidence – three schools, three sets of teachers, three sets of subjects, three sets of friends, all in three years.

When he was at the middle school – Amberfield, where Sophie and Adam were to go in due course and Sophie was to become head girl – he won a prize for 'Most Improved Pupil'. He received a large colourful book about wildlife with a tiger on the front.

Years later Sophie's friend, who was a lovely girl but perhaps not terribly bright, won the same prize. Forgetting at that moment that Michael had received it too, I blathered on about how when I was at school they gave that sort of prize to the child who worked hard but was actually rather thick. It was meant to be funny.

Even now, writing this, I cringe at the memory and wonder if Michael remembers this, too, and if it haunts him. I hope not. Perhaps he remembers a whole range of slights and jibes – meant to be jokes – that belittled and demeaned him. Did I spend all of his childhood coming out with this awful, ill-judged stuff, causing him to feel he was worthless and useless?

18 May 2008

Dear Michael,

We now seem to have lost Steve, the useless handyman. Your mother blames me (of course). Have to say he was hard work – and probably the dullest man I have ever met in my life. I just want someone to turn up, do the job and go, with payment at the end of the month or whatever. With Steve, he wanted to show me what he was doing for every little job, seemed to want to stop and have lunch with me, and needed to be told how well he was doing all the time. He's less an odd-job man, more a prima-donna ballerina.

Anyhow, I must have said or done something wrong on one of his recent blundering visits. I may have shown my irritation at his slowness. I may just have sighed theatrically when he asked for payment on the spot. Anyway, he's not returning my texts any more. I suppose it's possible he bored himself to death; he nearly did it to me.

I have had a bit of an interruption with my swimming on account of what feels like a trapped nerve in my neck. I've been staining the second half of the fence; a big job, some 900+ panels, and I made the tragic error of staining them with Autumn Brown instead of Harvest Brown, which was what I did the first half with; so do we have a fence in two shades of brown or do I stain it twice, once in each shade (or do I simply not care)? At present, with my neck, it's a mix of three shades – Harvest Brown, Autumn Brown and Whatever Was On It Before Brown. Your mother is not best pleased. There are pointed references to Frank Spencer.

I don't get much sympathy, I can tell you. I have not swum for the past couple of days. If I move my right arm in a circular motion, as if I were swimming, it sends shock waves up my neck. Your mother says not to do it. I have lain on the rug in the lounge and tried 'dry' breast stroke swimming to see if it hurts. It does. Your mother says it is ridiculous but, if you think about it, how else can you find out? Adam has been trying to get me to do the butterfly stroke. I haven't. I don't wish to become a YouTube sensation.

Now that the odd-job man – prima-donna Steve – has left us in the lurch, I have taken to calling traders from the freebie paper they push through the door on Thursdays. I know this is the fastest way to pay silly prices for poor service – I can't imagine anyone of any quality needing to advertise in a local free rag. All the downstairs sockets went off, no idea why. I checked the wiring in assorted sockets and plugs – they all seemed to be connected – and flipped switches off and on hopefully, to no avail. So we called out a local electrician.

He said he didn't do 'messy jobs' any more but that, as we were local and in trouble, he'd come round and take a look. I suspect the £27 per hour he wanted – £27! – had something to do with it too. Anyway, two days later he strolled up, looking like Keith Allen on a bad day, and said we'd need to replace some sort of electrical part on a board in the kitchen cupboard. Off he wandered, came back and fitted it and, hey presto, it was sorted. So, one hour's work, a part that he said cost £65. I got my cheque book out, ready to write a cheque for £92.

No! He wanted £156 and in cash. Um, I asked how that was broken down. Wasn't the part £65, he'd said? So, he explained, as if I were some sort of village idiot, that he had come round especially as a favour, had driven to get the part and come straight back and fitted it. He had, he said, given an excellent service and so had charged for four hours (instead of one) but then had discounted some of it because he'd got the part locally instead of having to drive into Ipswich. Simple.

My hand shaking with anger – I hate these sorts of rip-offs – I wrote a cheque for £92, left the name blank, and gave it to him, saying take it or leave it and, as matter of fact as I could, that I worked for the government (i.e. the implication I was someone official and very important – HMRC at least, MI5 more likely). He looked me up and down, no doubt taking in the *Doctor Who* T-shirt and jogging bottoms, before turning on his heel and marching out. Come back, prima-donna Steve, all is forgiven.

All for now,

Love

Dad

PS The prom saga continues. I will not bore you with the minutiæ of the full horror. Suffice to say that I have had a parent on the phone complaining about the cost of the ticket (£38). This from a woman who has never worked and has a trust fund. Apparently, the local state school are charging £25 so why weren't we? (Put darling Letitia in state school, why don't you?, and see how long she survives.)

On and on and on she goes until I snap and say I will give her a costs breakdown when I see her on Monday at the school (which will show that I am actually part-subsidising this wretched affair to keep the tickets at under £40). No offers to help. No support. Just endless freaking complaints. Honestly, if this were the US I'd go on a killing spree of parents at private schools. What is the matter with these freaks and weirdos?

Later, much later, when Michael and Niamh were a well-established couple, I remember all of us standing outside a cinema in Ipswich at some time or other with me making a joke at Adam's expense. It was meant to be a good-natured one that made Adam laugh. (I tend to joke about his inability with maths and he reciprocates with comments about my bald spot and the fact that, after eating, I usually find food remnants on my arms, down my shirt and in my hair.)

Niamh made a remark about 'an example of Iain's parenting skills'. I was not sure what to say and, in my mind at least, there then followed an awkward silence. It might just have been a passing comment but it set me thinking. How had Michael viewed me as a parent over the years? Was it my failings and shortcomings that loomed largest?

I had always thought we had a good relationship, full of jokes and banter. Michael always seemed to smile, laugh and take things in good spirit, I don't recall a raised eyebrow, a pulled face or shaken head at any time. It was the sort of relationship I would have wanted but had never had with my own father who, when I was a child of seven or eight, had brought his girlfriend into the house with my mother still there. My mother then had no real choice but to move out. I had such a rotten childhood that I had nothing to do with him after I left at eighteen. Over the years, I often feared I would fail to be a good father too.

June 2008

Hello Michael,

Three 'big' news stories . . .

The Prom

All in all, it seemed to go pretty well. The girls turned up in their finery in everything from a stretch limo to a tractor (tongue-in-cheek, theirs not mine). Most had boyfriends in tow who scrubbed up well enough and did not eff and blind or get drunk and vomit everywhere. There was some eating and some dancing (not by yours truly) and some photographs were taken by Hannah's mum, Angela, and sold on at cut-price rates. The teachers were all low-key but had a good time too. No one fought or argued or burst into tears which, with some thirty-odd teenage girls in attendance, must be some sort of record. Everyone came along except for a girl who has spots.

I could dwell on the negatives – only one girl (Farty Briony) actually thanked anyone for the work that was put in. Someone shouted, 'See you, Hagrid,' at me from amongst the crowd. That girl's mother cried off with a twisted ankle and the father dropped off the girl and then did a rapid three-point turn before hitting a bollard and driving off at speed. (If looks could kill I'd be dead. Still no idea why.) The woman that organised the event looked as though she were sucking lemons all night. But, when all is said and done, we did it for Sophie. She and Olivia and Leila enjoyed it. We did not let her down or embarrass her. We did our best. (But, in saying all that, I would not wish to do it again for all the world.)

The Picasso Incident

Saturday, I made the terrible mistake of what I think is called mis-fuelling, putting the wrong fuel in the car. Had this happened in my Espace and on a weekday when your mother was at work, I could probably have got it sorted no questions asked. As it was, your mother was off-duty and it was the Picasso; to make matters worse, she was in it at the time (we were nipping into Ipswich to have a look round, a.k.a. buy some clothes from H & M, etc.).

I knew what I had done – think blinding shaft of light – the moment I had filled the car up with £50 of petrol. I tried a double-bluff by driving away as if it were perfectly normal and we jerked and bunny-hopped as far as the Walton car wash when your mother turned to me and asked if I had put the wrong fuel in AGAIN. Again? How did she know? Anyhow, the Picasso is now ready to be towed to the garage on Monday and we are making do with the Espace.

Grandma's Party

As Grandma's 120th birthday is on Father's Day, we (your dear mother, Adam, Sophie and I) ran down there today (in the Espace). We had a pizza there for lunch and then played cards. It was okay. The problem with old people, generally, is that they do not eat very much. When you were small, and Nan died, we went down to sort Grandpa out (Grandad Terry and Granny were shooting craps in Las Vegas at that time and could not be disturbed). Grandpa ate so frugally that we were forever nipping out to the local shop, the burger place on the seafront and other assorted dives, to get food. It is the same with Grandma – we get cheesy pizzas (Lee would have been happy).

We then played Donkey and I did my usual sleight-of-hand at every opportunity (hold the Donkey on the bottom until you slip it to whoever you want). Funnily enough, Adam got the Donkey every single time. Eventually, they would not let me deal any more. If Grandma had not been present, I think there might have been a scene. We left about four thirty and got back at seven thirty; it always seems to take longer coming back. I don't know why. Can you maybe send a card or something? You should have the address – if not call your mother early this week. You do not have to spend any money (other than a stamp) but please acknowledge her existence. You can put Niamh's name on it if you wish.

Anyhow, that's all for now – see you on Father's Day!

Love

Dad

x

I have something of a reputation in the family when it comes to cars: running out of petrol and pranging them in multi-storey car parks, even mis-fuelling, are all par for the course. So too are my drives uphill in fourth gear and my emergency stops at roundabouts. No one bats an eyelid. Perhaps the best known, though, is the 'Do we have a shovel?' drama.

In brief, I was going to paint the ceilings in our loft rooms and bought a huge plastic tub – 'huge', 'plastic', 'tub' – of white matt paint, the biggest I could get from Homebase. It was too wide to tuck in behind the car seats even though the sides were pliable and bendy. I didn't want it sliding about in the boot so I put it on the back seat of the Picasso. All well and good so far (although, to be fair, you are no doubt ahead of me already, if not at the end of the story).

Driving back, I had to brake sharply by the local Tesco where some dim-witted fool stood back at the crossing, then lurched forward just as I was approaching. I duly performed a famed emergency stop rather than run him over – I wish I hadn't bothered – and the tub went flying, lid off, paint everywhere inside the car.

Hence the immortal words as I entered the kitchen, 'Do we have a shovel?' To cut a long story short – hours, we're talking – I got the worst of it up with a spade, managing to dump great thick dollops into bin bags (why are they so wretchedly flimsy?).

We then worked down through a range of spoons from the cutlery drawer and eventually to cloths and warm water. Even today you can still see where it was – I don't think it will ever come out or fade – but you have to be looking for it. We eventually passed the car on to Michael and told him to make out it was some sort of 'work of art'.

June 2008

Dear Michael,

We are close to the end of the school year now at both Amberfield and Ipswich (your mother goes on for about two more weeks, I think). It is sad that Sophie is now leaving Amberfield and our association with it finally ends after, what, fifteen years all-in?

Naturally, one girl's parents made a big show of presenting the school with some sports equipment at sports day and everyone clapped. It had never crossed my mind to do anything like that.

At the same time, another girl's parents – name escapes me – had obviously made some sort of hefty donation as a cup was presented in her name. I assume she was hoping for head girl. It should be called 'The Dah-De-Dah Cup Awarded for the Most Shameless Sucking Up'. I asked Sophie if we should have made some sort of donation from our extended overdraft facility but she pulled a face so I assume not.

I still remember that first day dropping Sophie off and, every day, her running into school, bag in one hand, the other clutching her straw hat on her head.

Sophie having Lucy Mac round for tea and telling her, for no obvious reason, I was going to punch her when taking her home. (She must have done something to 'set Sophie off'.)

Sophie, Lucy and Hope getting free after school one day before your mother got there and exploring the woods, cutting across the train track, etc. Huge drama!

Taking Sophie off for tennis tournaments; one at Bromley where some mother said Sophie looked like me (exchanged looks of mutual horror). The county tournament where I felt as though I were there to clean the toilets given the way everyone spoke to me. The things I have had to put up with through gritted teeth for Sophie.

Netball for the county and overhearing one father say, after Sophie had scored yet another goal, that his side might have won if it hadn't been for 'the big girl'. I wanted to nudge him and say, 'That's my big girl.'

Nick telling me that Wendy [Lucy Mac's mum] had terminal cancer as we stood waiting for the girls outside the music room. I knew at that point I should have hugged him but my usual hopelessness with all things emotional took over and I just stood there mumbling and trying not to cry. As ever, I must have looked totally heartless. Your mother says my 'at ease' face looks like a murderer's. As she says I also have a peculiar smile that does not suit my face, I am slightly stuck as to know what expression to strike at any given moment. At that one, it should have been utter sadness.

Wendy's funeral with your dear mother, Sophie and Olivia. Lucy trying to make a speech and breaking down. I wanted to stand up and shout, 'Go on, Lucy, you can do it.' As always, my nerve failed me. A sad day. Jackson – maybe too young to take it all in – said a few words; not a dry eye in sight.

Sophie getting head girl. I had to go and pick her up for something or other on the morning it was announced. There were five of them up for it. I thought Sophie would get it but did not want to say so in advance. Had she not got it, I would have been blamed. She came out, matter-of-factly telling me, and I nodded and said that was good. I could not speak until we got into the car.

I also remember Adam first going there when he was five – and he would always seem happy when I dropped him off in the classroom but would have a huge fit as I left. Mrs Boyd having to wrestle him to the ground whilst I made my escape.

I remember taking Adam and his friend Lou to *Robot Wars* at the Wolsey Theatre. I bought them both a robot toy at the interval. Lou chose first. Then Adam. Lou then wanted Adam's robot when we sat down. Adam swapped round. For the rest of the second half, Lou kept casting envious glances at his old toy, now Adam's. Cue various whining noises and 'Yours is really good, Adam' comments (evidently, Lou really wanted both toys for himself). After the show, Lou wanted Adam to swap back. Adam refused (he had clearly had enough too). We drove Lou home in silence apart from a faint whimpering noise. Happy days.

I was thinking, maybe if you are free over the next week or two, you could possibly come down and see Adam. I will pay for the car or train, etc. You could maybe see a film together at Ipswich. He will be a little spare until your mother breaks up. Let us know?

Love

Dad

x

PS We need to make some arrangements for Bernard whilst we are away in Orlando. Can Niamh's folks have him? I remember Niamh telling me that one of them does dog-sitting? I cannot bear to think of Bernard in a kennels. The constant barking would upset him. He is a sensitive fellow; it's like walking on eggshells at times.

Is there any defence to the charge that I made Michael what he became? I might well have been hopeless with showing emotions and, indeed, talking to him and listening to his thoughts – after all, letters, emails and texts are all ways of keeping emotional stuff at arm's length. (And Michael kept himself to himself anyway, other than the odd drawing and card.) But I'd say I was always there, above and beyond taking him to school and back and playing about in the evening. I was present for every birthday, the parties when he was younger and what have you as he got older. I remember taking him and twelve or so of his friends to an Ipswich Town football match. There was paintballing too. I took two weeks off at Christmas to spend time together as a family. We went to *The Sooty Show* in London for many years, then pantos and other shows, *The Snowman*, *Chitty Chitty Bang Bang* at the Palladium and more.

I went to sports days and parents' evenings and lots of musical evenings where little girls pranced and preened and big strapping lads bellowed out songs horribly out of tune. Dear God, the endless bilge I've had to sit through and smile. A version of Elton John's 'Candle In The Wind' lingered long in the memory as the three worst minutes of my life until, at a later concert for one of the other children, we had to listen to some tone-deaf lump grunt his way through Snow Patrol's 'Run'. (If only we could have.)

As Michael got older, I stood in the wind every week as he did his karate in the local school gym; fifty to sixty pairs of bare feet in an enclosed space can be overpowering if you walk in unawares. I sat in the car in damp and rainy weather on many Sundays as he played football for the local village team. Michael was self-conscious and didn't like to be watched – he'd suggest I stayed in the car, the parking area being a safe distance away. We went to football – Ipswich Town matches home and away, England at Wembley. We even took him out of school one day to go to Manchester United at Old Trafford – our cover blown to the school and teachers when we walked in front of the Sky TV cameras without realising it.

People these days seem to equate love with huge expressions of physical affection. I've never been someone who instinctively hugs and kisses, even those who are nearest and dearest to me. I am certainly not a hugger of friends, colleagues and passing acquaintances: it is all too Princess Diana.

Fortunately, I have been told over the years, by my nearest and dearest, that I have an imposing presence and that my face – even when I'm thinking benign thoughts about an upcoming choice of puddings – suggests I am about to kill somebody. So I'm not someone who you would normally want to hug in case it ended in attempted murder or death. The whole hugging and kissing thing makes me go all hot. Neither can I talk about feelings. I can write them down well enough, charting events, working out ideas, flexing my humour muscles even, but face-to-face, the wet and soggy stuff? Heaven above, I'd have to cover my face with my hands. But I believe I did my best in my own peculiar way. Is that enough?

July 2008

Hello Michael,

We are all back at home all day long for the whole summer, Orlando excluding, God help us. It seems strange you not being here but your permanent presence would no doubt add to the general melee. I have to shut the loft door sometimes so I can hear myself think – Sophie's whisper is like a foghorn three floors up. And when a squabble breaks out it's like World War III.

It does not help that I am doing 'double-work'. July is always a pain as I have to write not only July's material but August's as well for when we are away. The newsletters are easy enough as most of that is timeless but to write newsy emails a month beforehand is a nightmare in waiting – a couple of years back I took to writing newsy emails a few days in advance in case I was taken ill one day. I made some comments about holidaying somewhere: of course, I then forgot all about it and it went out the day after a disaster there.

I am also having problems with my phone. God, I hate the mobile company. Whenever you have a problem, you speak to some fellow in India. I know it's probably not PC to say so, and I accept his English is way better than my Indian, but if someone works in telephone sales, they need to be understood, surely. We started off badly, with him asking if he could call me 'Ann'. I said, 'You can call me what you want as long as you fix my wretched phone.' Needless to say, he didn't and, thirty-five minutes, and four different conversations later, I raised my voice to the woman on the other end of the line and said the word 'bloody'. Hey presto, she cut me off on the spot.

Lulu is to have Bernard whilst we are away. We are pleased about that as they are a normal family with a dog and Bernard should just fit in nicely. We were not keen on kennels – when we had Carmel, she went into a cattery for a week whilst we went to Cornwall and when we came out she sat with her back to us for a good fortnight. I dread to think what Bernard would be like as he is a much fussier fellow.

Holiday-wise, are you ready? We fly from Gatwick at about noon on the Sunday so we will leave here at 6 a.m. to allow plenty of time to get there. We should land at Orlando at about 4 p.m. (five hours behind) and be in the villa by about 5.30; but note it will feel like 10.30 and we will have been up since 5 a.m. We will sleep in the next morning to catch up.

Probably best not to say too much to Niamh about the mini-coach hoo-hah if she is not a good traveller. Needless to say, I won't be eating fish before we set off this year so we can, hopefully, avoid the vomit stops and the rush to the WC when we arrive so I can bin my clothes. No coach this year, I will drive us.

Do you and Niamh want to come over Sunday evening so we can just run through the rest of the Orlando stuff and tickets and what have you? We can get a Chinese and have it round the table; do you eat Chinese still? Your mother says you prefer vegetarian food more these days. Is that principle or personal preference? Anyway, you can have a bowl of noodles and seaweed although they won't put much meat on your bones. Talk to your dear mother.

Love

Dad

PS Lulu's Dad is something big in rubbish tips and was asked to go on *The Secret Millionaire* but refused. I imagine he wants to keep the million quiet. Someone else told me recently that the guy who owns that big car breaker's yard at Bramford is a millionaire. I am obviously in the wrong job. All I have is a big overdraft. These days, you get money by getting your hands dirty because no one else wants to do it. When I started writing back in 1987, I was a freak – no one really did it. Now, everyone with online access is a writer and they do it all for free. Nightmare.

The truth is that I really don't know whether Michael's troubles, which were soon to be made all too apparent to us, were down to me or to him or maybe a mixture of both or something else completely. If you judge a father by how many times they say 'I love you' and how often they hug you, then I am a complete and utter failure.

But, as indicated, I was an ever-present dad. I did not work in London every day, leaving at 6 a.m. and arriving home exhausted at 10 p.m. after the children had gone to bed. I did not go to pubs drinking on Friday and Saturday nights. I did not disappear at weekends fishing or motorbiking, doing whatever it is that real men do. I always put my children before myself. I would step in front of the proverbial big red bus for them.

Later, when Michael and I talked a little, and we did talk on occasions, he said that what happened was nothing to do with us,

Tracey and me or the family: we had not contributed to his down-fall. Of course that didn't stop us seeking to uncover the root of the problem and whether we were to blame for it.

He might have been telling the truth. Perhaps he was being kind or didn't really know. I'm not sure but, looking back, I seem to have been determined, despite the growing signs and then the evidence, to ignore all of it and just keep talking and writing nonsense. Whether I was a good or a bad dad, there is little doubt that I was a stupid one.

21 September 2008

Michael,

We all seem to be back into our normal grooves again at last although I still seem to be playing catch-up with the newsletters (think domino-effect). Your mother has the little ones this time round; the poo and wee brigade. Sophie and Adam are back at Ipswich (if you were Maitland Major and Adam is Maitland Minor, what is Sophie? We've suggested Maitland Mental). Sophie has already started partying with assorted posh boys and pony girls; how long she and Lee will keep going I would not like to say. He is very much a Tizer and cheese puffs kind of lad. We like him, though. If they are still together, we may invite him on next year's holiday. Olivia is now at Colchester and I think Megan has long gone. We may do Spain, a beach villa?

Your dear mother has now seen *Mamma Mia* five times with assorted friends. (I refuse to go having seen a clip of Pierce Brosnan's singing in it on Anglia Television.) I think it's going to be a close-run thing – whether they stop showing it first or your mother runs out of friends. I fear she may win this one. She has the scent of blood in her nostrils.

I have, under pressure from your dear mother, made a small, one-off – note small, note one-off – transfer into your bank account. This is simply to cover you up to when you get your grant money in (or whatever they call it these days). Do not race to your nearest cashpoint: the amount is small and designed to last you a week or two, no more. It may be a little more than you need. I err on the generous side. Some fathers would say that you can give back what you do not use. I know better than to ask.

Your mother is convinced that you will, given time and encouragement (pointed look at yours truly), prove to be a successful artist. I am less convinced. Your mother looks at your various efforts and sees genius. I tend to see lumps and daubs. Of course, that weird shop at Downtown Disney with the alien-thing drawings did not help matters. It simply excited your mother as the work was, and I quote, 'almost the same as Michael's'. I imagine one serial killer's work is much like another's when all is said and done.

All I ask of you is that you work hard over this year and next and try to get a decent degree that you can use to get

a job. You may well be the next Damien Hirst or Tracey
Emin – your bedroom on holiday bore a striking resemblance to her 'masterpiece' – but this is something you need
to progress in your spare time; you cannot sit around for
years like Van Gogh waiting to be discovered (not on my
money anyway). Get some sort of job to pay your way and
do the fancy stuff in the evening and weekends. Then, when
you are discovered you can glue your ear back on and live
happily ever after.

I also think you could do with building yourself up a
bit. This veggie business has left you looking rather
skinny. You and Niamh both. It's good that you are nice
and slim but I think you have to be careful not to take
things too far. Niamh keeling over is something of a
heads-up.

What are Niamh's plans? This degree she's doing – what
is it, medieval fabric-making – sounds fascinating but is it
going to get her a job at Greggs? Many of these clever-dick
degrees they have these days are not going to get anyone
anywhere. When I was young, you had universities and
proper subjects and only clever boys and girls went there.
They had polytechnics for those who were 'less academic'. It
all then became a free-for-all with Stoke Poly, Grimsby
Asylum and the Cleethorpes Home for Escaped Raving
Lunatics all becoming 'universities' and acting like they
were Oxford and Cambridge. They all do wacky degrees
that no employer wants – The Beatles, *Doctor Who*, the Role

of Alvin & The Chipmunks in a Multi-Ethnic Society. Do something – both of you – that can be used in everyday practical life.

All for now, go check that cash machine. We will need to give some thought soon to birthdays, yours and Adam's, so maybe liaise with your mother. We are due to see Granny next Sunday; some castle in Kent (not Hever for a change) and I will drop you a line when I get back. Maybe you and Niamh could come down and join us some time. Or at least come over and see her when she comes up the weekend before Christmas (20th, I think).

Love

Dad

x

PS If/when you get into conversation with Sophie, avoid the whole GCSE thing. We thought she did just fine. She was expecting As galore. Other girls did better. All very much a sore point even now.

We – the five of us, plus Niamh – spent three weeks in Orlando in the summer of 2008, doing the rounds of the Disney and Universal theme parks. It went well and we had a good time – or at least I thought we did (although Michael and Niamh chose not to come with us on the Orlando trip in 2010 because, they said, of the flight times and the heat). But my two main memories of the trip are telling. They were the first real suggestions that all was not as it should have been.

One features Niamh who fainted in the heat during some sort of *Indiana Jones*-type show. Looking back, she was not the same-sized girl we had first met in 2007 and, as time passed, Tracey and I wondered if she had gone on a diet and had encouraged Michael to do the same – a diet that, in Michael's case, he had taken to excess.

The other, apparently inconsequential, memory is of Michael not wanting to eat any of the Chinese take-out we had ordered and had been delivered to the villa one night later in the holiday. I remember shouting something at him along the lines of 'Why not just stop eating altogether and go straight to hospital?' I had no conscious idea at this stage that anything was particularly wrong but was clearly irritated by what I saw as Michael's endless fussiness about eating during the trip. Evidently, he was not really eating much at all and at some level I had spotted that but had not absorbed its full significance. I don't think any of us, other than Michael and Niamh, had.

September 2008

Michael,

We 'braved the Sunday crowds' (as Grandpa used to say, as if we were storming the beaches of Normandy) and had a lovely day out with Granny at Leeds Castle (for a change). I don't suppose you remember Grandpa much? Great Grandpa to you, really. You'll have seen the photo I have of him in my room? The one where, for reasons best known to himself, he has a cereal bowl upside down on his head. I think he was trying to amuse Sophie when she was in her high-chair.

It's strange to think that, just twelve years or so after his death, there are probably no more than a handful of people at most, if any really, other than some of us, who ever think of him. I Googled 'Charles Gayther' and 'Edna Gayther' plus 'West Norwood' the other day. Nothing came up. It's as if they never existed. I remember them, not every day but fairly often, and they are always happy thoughts. A quick history lesson (in case I drop down dead tomorrow and you then decide you wanted to know about your family line).

Grandpa, Charles Gayther, born Southport, 1907. Father, hairdresser, mother Charlotte (hence, Charles coming down the family line). Two brothers, Harold (didn't like), Wallace (died young). Moved to Nottingham in 1912 due to some sort of hairdressing scandal. The 'Great Southport Syrup of Figs Scandal 1912' maybe.

Met Edna, Nan, in Nottingham. Sister, Queenie. Mother, can't remember, but lived until she was ninety-two (very impressive in the 1960s). Ran an offal shop. Father left when young and had another family (Granny met them a year or two back via some ancestry site – now in Australia and one is called Tegan). The father was a Winston

Churchill lookalike in the war. Some talk of him 'standing in' for the great man at events. Most likely did impressions for money outside pubs.

Moved to London for work in late 1930s. Granny, my mother, born 1935. Roger born 1945. Roger died of meningitis when he was twenty. I remember him clearly. He had an electric guitar and did magic tricks. I recall sitting outside a hospital with green railings. They packed him in ice. Tragic. Grandpa went to work the next day. No one spoke to him. It was the only time in his life he lost his stammer.

Grandpa was a talented musician and won various *Melody Maker* awards in the thirties. Could either have been a full-time musician or get 'a proper job' and play semi-pro. He played safe (for the family) and I think he regretted it at times. It's what encouraged me to be a writer – not that I expected a life of 'Say Aloe to a Cleaner Bowel' to be my bread and butter. Anyhow, Grandpa ended up working in factories all his life. Nan worked for Freemans, a catalogue company. No dukes and duchesses in our line, I'm afraid.

They moved down to Littlehampton in 1975; sea air for Nan's emphysema. I used to stay there for much of the school holidays; fairly ghastly home life. I was an only child, my parents divorcing when I was eight. My father had a much younger wife as close to my age as his. My mother had a much older husband who lived with his mother until he was fifty. I spent Monday to Thursday at my father's, Friday to Sunday at my mother's. So it was all a bit *Addams Family**. Nan died in 1988, the year my mother and her next husband, Terry, moved nearby. Grandpa died in 1996. Sad times.

Anyway, I digress. The joys of Leeds Castle! I had thought it was where they filmed *Doctor Who* (Jon Pertwee, Jo, Bessie, waving at camera etc.) and raved about it all the way down until we arrived and I realised it wasn't. Anyway, we did the usual – inside, lunch, outside – and Sophie said 'penis' over pudding. We left about four so Granny could get back ('to avoid the traffic', as Grandpa would put it). We have two carefully wrapped presents, one for you and one for Adam, and we will give you yours when we see you. Please remember to thank Granny – maybe a handmade card with something appropriate for a granny on it? (No blood and guts, please.) That would be nice.

Love

Dad

x

PS Adam is attempting the violin. God, it's awful. Think nails on a blackboard. It starts. The dog sits bolt upright. It continues for a few moments, laboured and repetitive. It stops. We all hold our breath. The dog slumps back down. It starts again. The dog sits bolt upright; and so it goes, round and round.

*The Addams Family, for those of a younger generation, was a macabre bunch of assorted freaks and ghouls; much like some members of my own family as a child. I remember sitting in a car, my father and mother in the front, me and his girlfriend in the back, outside my nan and grandpa's house. I was told by my father that I had to say, if either grandparent asked, that his now living-with-us girlfriend sitting next to me was, in fact, my teacher who was lodging with us for a while as she had nowhere else to stay. I would have been about seven when I was primed for that pretence. There were many other horrors to come.

9 November 2008

Dear Michael,

We have had an unfortunate day today and your mother is in something of a mood with me. I am relying on you to give her a call on some pretext and sing my praises.

It started when the four of us went to the Suffolk food hall and bumped into some work colleagues of your mother in the café. We had to sit with them (groan). I am always expected, on such occasions, to look smart (I had last night's dinner T-shirt on plus gardening shoes without laces), to be bright and cheery (not really my thing) and not to say anything that would offend anyone (as if). I thought I had got away with it but apparently I made a *faux pas* when they talked about getting a puppy. I said I'd seen a programme where dogs left on their own all day went mad and banged their heads against the walls. I thought I was being mildly amusing but as they'd said they would have to leave it at home all day, popping back at lunchtimes only, I had apparently caused some offence. Your mother said it sounded as though I were 'having a go' at them.

It then got worse when we went to the carpet store up at B & Q as I'd been talked into replacing Adam's carpet (it still has that big purple stain). Your mother had decided that Adam should have the same sort of carpet as Sophie; a sort of brown and white ridged thing that 'doesn't show the dirt'. We were pounced on within seconds by some hard-faced woman in a suit who asked who the carpet was for. I was tiring badly in the charm stakes at this point and said something untoward, like 'Well, Adam is having it, my wife is choosing it and I am paying for it.' Sophie and Adam laughed but your mother did not. The saleswoman looked bemused. It was a little like the parents' evening when a new teacher asked what Adam was good at. I said something along the lines of 'We don't know, we're still searching.' The teacher looked at me as if I were mad. Anyway, a carpet was duly chosen and off we went, all of us trying to avoid your mother's black looks.

We then had to go to Nacton Shores for Adam for some fossil project or other. It was all getting rather fraught at this stage so I dropped off your mother and Adam and took Sophie home to do some homework (i.e. text her friends all afternoon), saying I would go back and collect your mother and Adam. I went straight back knowing that if your mother were kept waiting I'd be for it. Anyway, an hour and a half later – now dark and really quite spooky – your mother and Adam appeared, your mother having fallen over and trodden in something. We travelled home in near silence and your mother has not really spoken to me since. Call her please – now.

Love

Dad

PS That Nacton Shores car park is a funny place. In the space of ninety minutes, four middle-aged men turned up there in succession on their own, two in cars, two on foot. They all disappeared for a few minutes at a time, then reappeared and went away again. They all looked at me quite pointedly. I just smiled vaguely at them – your mother says it's polite – and carried on reading my book.

Digressing slightly to end the year on a cheerful note, I was, in my younger days, something of a magnet to gay men (hard to believe now when I catch sight of this bloated wreck in an unexpected mirror). I was regularly offered drinks in bars and propositioned by men when playing snooker.

I was even, on one memorable occasion, picked up by a man who stopped in his car and asked me for directions. In my teenage naivety, I offered to get into the car – he was going my way – to show him where he wanted to go. We ended up in some woods in a kind of *Carry On* scene, with me playing the Barbara Windsor role while being chased by Sid James. *Carry On Up the Khyber*, I think it was.

Anyway, sitting in what was, and I believe still is, a meeting place for homosexual chaps, it was good to see that I had not lost it. My dear wife would be surprised to learn I'd had it in the first place. Still, we end 2008, somewhat improbably, with me as a gay icon.

2009

We start the year with everything appearing to be much the same as it had ever been. I was still scribbling health, wealth and happiness articles although – seeing the writing on the wall (the free-of-charge writing on the internet, really) – I was moving into property matters which, as the years passed, proved a more reliable source of income. Tracey was still working at the local primary school and enjoying it.

Our children's lives were changing as they were growing up. Sophie was doing A levels – again, expectations were high, from Sophie anyway. She was hoping to get three As if not three A*s before being carried off shoulder high to university. Adam was due to move up to his senior school soon and we were unsure which school, if any, would be best for him.

As for Michael, he was now entering his own private Hell, stressed and anxious while trying, at least to us and the wider world, to convey an impression that all was well. The year 2009 was a turning point and an opportunity for us to see that all was not well and to take steps to stop Michael going into freefall. To say we failed miserably is an understatement.

11 January 2009

Dear Michael,

There is not too much to report in the way of news. Niamh mentioned in passing that you spend every day in the Odeon – I hope that was a joke or at least is not literally true; I hope you are working hard and getting the grades you need to get a decent degree. When I was at school, in black and white days, few people did A levels let alone a degree – a degree was something really special. Nowadays, everyone seems to have one so do try to get the highest grade that you can to give you the best possible chance of what people call 'a job'.

Talking cinemas, I've just been reading the Top 10 box office movies. When I was your age, I'd have seen all of them. These days, I have seen four and two of those I slept through. I saw *Indiana Jones and the Crystal Skull* (not sure getting in a fridge would save you from a nuclear blast) and *Quantum of Solace* (way too nasty-violent for a 12). I slept through *Wall-E* and *Kung Fu Panda*; or at least most of them anyway.

I always remember the Christmas Eve films – I invariably slept through all of them (I was winding down for Christmas). I recall *The Prince of Egypt* when we had Carl and Lauren; I awoke at one point to see the four of you all watching me. I dread to think what woke me up. Not my surround-sound snoring, I hope.

The two most memorable films I didn't see this year were *Mamma Mia* and *Hancock*. I think your dear mother stretched various friendships to breaking point with *Mamma Mia* and came close to dragging people off the street to see it with her. *Hancock* was a great disappointment. When I first heard the title, I assumed it was about the lad himself. Then I discovered it was starring Will Smith – stone me, a great actor but hard to see him portraying Tony Hancock.

I forgot to say that we are going to have a beach holiday this year, probably in Spain. No idea where. First two weeks of August most likely. You and Niamh are welcome to come; as it is an easyJet job I am happy to pay for your flights if we can get sorted and book early. Sophie and, I think, Lee are coming along so let me know asap and I will start looking at places and villas. We will try to get somewhere within walking distance of a beach and with one or two places to visit so we can have a beach day and a something-else day and a beach day, etc. Lee says they have good waterparks there so I will see if we can get ourselves based near to one. (I'm not sure he can actually swim so his enthusiasm beats me.)

Love

Dad

Michael was now spending most of his days in the cinema. There was an Odeon halfway between where he lived and where he was doing his degree. He loved routine, and sitting cocooned in the dark, transported to another world, was the easiest way for him to hide from the world that made him feel so anxious. Work, money, bills, taking responsibility, were all threatening issues for him. Sitting in a cinema for hours at a stretch allowed him to feel safe.

Two memories come to me. One was that time when Michael was doing his A levels and someone said something nasty about his appearance. Then, chatting with Tracey about how he was getting on at school, he had confided that he wished he was young again: he didn't really want to grow up. Tracey responded by saying that was a perfectly normal thought. She mentioned it to me as we talked over a pub lunch a few days later but we didn't think much of it – it was just a transient moment, a passing feeling that many young people must have from time to time as work and responsibilities start pressing in. Now it is telling.

The other memory is from a year or two later. Michael sent me a birthday card of the sort that would have been bought by a young child, perhaps of nine or less. 'To Daddy' at the top and a cartoon spaceman on the front. There might even have been a 'Best Daddy' badge to wear. I was not sure how to take it. I thought it was odd at the time but laughed it off as a joke. Maybe it was. Now I'm not so sure. Maybe somewhere, deep down, it was a cry for help. If it was, I wasn't listening.

1 February 2009

Dear ITFC Superfan,

You will find, attached, a photo from the *Evening Star* sports pages. As you will see, it is of the Ipswich Town crowd celebrating wildly when Alex Bruce got the goal against Chelsea. Look closely, and you will see me and Adam jumping up joyfully with our arms in the air. You, between us, are sitting there as though you were doing Sudoku on the bus to Bury St Edmunds. Did you not notice the goal?

It's a shame you could not have come down with us earlier when we went to the *Doctor Who* shop. There was a massive queue to meet David Morrissey and I did not think we would get autographs, then across from East Ham to Fulham Broadway in time for the match. We only did because I mentioned to the shop owner that we were Ipswich supporters going to the football and she pulled us out and sent us to the front of the queue. I think she – or maybe David Morrissey – dislikes Chelsea or maybe she just felt sorry for us.

He seemed a nice guy. I think it was his first signing. We had the usual stilted conversation (I never know what to say on such occasions but am always determined to act normal and not create the impression I am a middle-aged *Doctor Who* fan who still lives with his mother). Me: I read in the local paper that you got married in Suffolk. Him: Yes.

Me: On the pier at Southwold. Him: That's right. Me: We like Southwold. Him: It's nice.

I am not a great conversationalist. (Your mother says I am incapable of small-talk, only droning on or shouting at people.) It was the same when we met Ian Lavender at Bressingham – Pike from *Dad's Army*? Me: Have you been here before? Pike: To Bressingham? Me: Yes. Pike: No. End of conversation. That, of course, was the day when, after meeting Jimmy Perry (the writer), Adam walked up to his wife, lifted her skirt and put his head inside. Cue embarrassed laughter all round. Fortunately, they found it funny. Your mother was mortified. Apparently, it was my fault for 'encouraging him'.

Do you get a half-term on your course? I cannot remember. If you do, we must try and have a get-together and maybe go somewhere different for a change. Not a good time of year outdoor-wise. We need to do something inside where we can just sit there. A circus maybe? Any ideas?

Love

Dad

x

PS What was that all about with your train ticket? I didn't catch what the railway man was saying. You had to wait until seven thirty as it was a special-priced ticket? I gave you £70 for the ticket so if you've been given a £10 special by the man behind the desk at Norwich, has he pocketed the difference? You need to go and ask. Otherwise, we've been scammed for £60. Let me know.

Michael and I had – still have to a degree – a way of spending time together without actually talking about anything, what we've done, what we're doing, let alone any sort of conversation about feelings, hopes and fears or anything of an emotional nature. We could quite easily meet up and go to a football match – albeit rarely by 2009 – and go home with the most intimate conversation being 'Do you want a matchday programme?' (I'd be buying it, naturally.)

By early 2009 cracks were developing in our relationship. I had gone down to London early in the day, with Adam, for that signing with actor David Morrissey at the *Doctor Who* shop. We then made our way to Stamford Bridge for the FA Cup tie between Chelsea and Ipswich Town. Michael met us there. He could easily have spent the day with us but just came down for the match and went straight back to Norwich again on the train. Why? Because, I realise now, it meant he could avoid the issue of breakfast, lunch and dinner.

Thinking back, I remember going to see an England match at Wembley with Michael (but not Adam as it was a school night) in what must have been 2007. We drove down and had some tea first at South Mimms services – I ate a proper meal, sausages, chips or whatever – while Michael said he wasn't hungry. I never gave it much thought at the time but it has more significance now. Even then, he wasn't eating properly, I just never really noticed.

Michael had ummed and aahed about joining us for the Ipswich v Chelsea match, citing the costs, and I had told him to buy a return train ticket from Norwich to London and I'd pay. Later, when we went to see him back on the train to Norwich, he said he had to wait for the one after the next as that was the one stated on his ticket. I took it to the ticket office to ask if he could get the earlier train and the response was no: this was a special priced ticket at just a tenner and the traveller had to journey in and out on a particular train. Michael said he had been ripped off by whoever had sold him the ticket. I suggested he went and got the money back. It was not mentioned again.

February 2009

Dear International Playboy,

Valentine's Day is fast approaching and I think, now that you have been with Niamh for quite some time, it's about time we talked 'women'. Having been with your dear mother for almost thirty endless years, I have some ideas about how best to handle them. They can be tricky, especially at this time of year when it is so easy to get things wrong. Here's my advice.

Hair – always be alert to a change in hairstyle or colour. You don't need to know the type of hairstyle or the shade of colour involved, you just need to spot it immediately (you don't get a second chance). The inevitable question that follows, 'Do you like it?', is trickier than it sounds. There is only one answer, 'Yes', but do not be too enthusiastic as it may be taken that you did not like the old hairstyle (she may switch back soon).

It's generally wise to make encouraging noises rather than saying what it is you like about the new hairstyle/ colour (not always easy if you cannot quite tell how it's different). Additional comments are always fraught with danger. The fallout from a perfectly simple 'It makes you look years younger' or 'It makes your face look slimmer' can be frightful, however well meant.

There will, now and then, be times when a woman will not like her hairstyle. You will know this because she will come into the house at some speed and head straight to the bathroom. On these occasions, it's generally best to keep out of the way as best you can and not say, 'Oh dear,' (or anything stronger) when you see her. As often as not, the hairstyle/colour will look perfectly fine to you and you will not know what all the fuss is about. It may not look any different to you. Do not say this. It is an argument you cannot win. You just have to let things run their course. A shed is useful on such occasions.

Eyes – do you know Niamh's eye colour? You need to. Do be aware that women never have 'blue' or 'brown' eyes. It can never be as simple or as straightforward as that. Your mother, for example, has hazelnut eyes with flecks of mint green. God forbid I should ever forget the fine detail. Take note.

Figure – no woman is entirely happy with all aspects of their figure. You need to find out, by listening carefully, which bits and bobs are considered satisfactory and which are not. This can be a time-consuming and thankless process and there are no shortcuts; you have to put in the hours in clothes shops. Clearly, you can praise the good bits to the rooftops. You never mention the bad bits (even though they probably look perfectly serviceable to you).

Referring again to your dear mother – for I have no other significant point of reference – I know, from hard-won experience, that she thinks she has long arms, a short waist and 'average' length legs and that she does not like the way she walks. This, when written down, suggests more than a passing resemblance to an orangutan but I think you'll agree this is a little harsh.

Feet – feet are funny things. To you and me, they are just there doing what they do, manoeuvring the remote control towards you so you can change channels, pushing the dog off the sofa when you want to lie down, and so on. Not with women. To them, feet are either things of great beauty or great ugliness; there never seems to be any in-between.

Some women tend to think they have beautiful feet and are constantly fiddling with them, taking varnish on and off, and wearing shoes that show them off to great effect. Others are embarrassed by them, usually because they are great hulking things best suited to plimsolls.

I have a system that allows you to identify what's what – check the shoe size. Up to about five or six and it's a thumbs-up feet-wise. Up at the nines and tens, it's a thumbs-down. In between? Move to the next system check – do they fancy up their feet with nail varnish and all of that? It's usually a thumbs-up but, please note, varnish can be applied to disguise perceived-to-be ugly feet. Check the footwear – are the feet covered up? It's another clue.

So there you have it – a short but invaluable guide to women and how they think and feel about themselves. You can use this to offer compliments at the right time, such as 'That top will go well with your hazelnut and mint-green eyes' or 'That dress will show off your feet to best effect.' Your mother always gives me an incredulous look when I come out with comments like these. I don't think she can believe how thoughtful and attentive I am.

With love

Dad

PS Bad weather – it's tempting to buy something sensible like wellington boots or a spade for Valentine's Day. Don't. I have been there, done that, got the bloodied T-shirt. You can say that they're worth keeping in the boot of the car in case you need to dig yourself out of the snow as much as you like – it does not help one bit. Trust me. Buy perfume, it's a safe bet.

Women, eh? I still have no idea what it's all about.

February 2009

Dear Michael,

The four of us tried that Thai restaurant. I'd not recommend it. We arrived early at about six for one reason or another and, not knowing what to order, we had the set menu for four – starter, main course, a pud and a tea or coffee. Simple – so we thought.

All went well up to about seven thirty. We were the only people there and had three or four of the staff faffing around us constantly. I quite liked that. Between seven thirty and seven forty-five, just as we were finishing the main course, the whole restaurant filled up, one end to the other.

No problem, we thought, we just have the pudding and the tea or coffee to go – we'd be done in half an hour. One and a half hours later, we left. We got a new waitress between the main course and the pudding; it went well to start with as I thought she was winking at me (turns out she had some sort of blinking, obsessive-compulsive thing going on, more fool me for winking back). Anyway, she told us that, as part of the set menu, we could EITHER have ice cream (the range of puddings being vanilla ice cream or vanilla ice cream with sprinkles) OR a hot drink (tea or coffee). Not what it said on the menu, but still, we went with the ice cream with sprinkles (Sophie and Adam hushing me down to avoid embarrassment).

Some twenty minutes later, at the point at which we were all staring into space with nothing left to say, we get the ice cream; two small portions (no sprinkles) and two spoons for the four of us. Again, Sophie and Adam shushed me down before I could say anything. I'd just about had it by this point I can tell you especially as someone – I think it was Sophie 'Always Calm' Maitland – said the word 'childish'. As I explained, I'm not childish. I am forty-seven and I don't want to share. I just want an ice cream with sprinkles of my own.

As we were finishing, the waitress came back, twitching and blinking – 'Very sorry,' she said, she had misread the menu. Ah, we thought, two more ice creams (with sprinkles this time?) are on their way. Not so, apparently, we were entitled to tea or coffee AS WELL. So, Adam declining the offer, we asked for two coffees (Sophie and me) and one tea (your dear mother).

No such luck – as with the ice cream, no sprinkles, we could have two drinks, one tea and one coffee or two teas or two coffees but not two coffees and one tea despite the fact that this was a set meal for four and I've never yet had a set meal for four where you've had to share two (small) ice creams (no sprinkles) and two hot drinks. Anyway, by this time I was muttering and mumbling loudly whilst Sophie and Adam talked over the top of me as if it were all perfectly normal.

Another wait and, eventually, we get one tea and one coffee; small cups, no refills. At this stage, we were all getting tense and starting to snipe away at each other. I wanted to say something to the manager. After all, if you walked into a pub and ordered, say, eight G & Ts and paid whatever that costs and you were given two (with straws) you'd say something – in fact, do that to a hairy docker in Felixstowe and you'd get a broken nose for it. Sophie and Adam wanted me to be quiet. Your mother said nothing (she does this meditation thing where she relaxes by thinking she is somewhere else; back home, most likely). She sat there humming. I sat there simmering.

Eventually, when we had all calmed down, I waved the owner over to pay the bill. I did explain slowly and carefully that, having ordered a set menu for FOUR, I expected FOUR ice creams (with sprinkles if we bloody well asked for them) and FOUR hot drinks. Naturally enough, it was at this point that his English failed completely and he smiled vacantly at me (an old trick that fools nobody – he regained his grasp of English three minutes later when I tried to press the 'No' tip on the credit-card machine).

Anyway, the long and the short of it was that we spent two and a half hours of our life there, for very average food, for more than £100 and we are still owed for two ice creams and two hot drinks, plus some sprinkles. If the children had not been with us I'd have been tempted to press my bare fat backside against the window as I left in protest.

Anyhow, that's all that's been happening lately – other than that we are all well and tickety-boo and we hope you are too.

Love

Dad

PS Talking Thai, it reminds me that many years ago, when as a boy I used to spend the summers at Nan and Grandpa's in West Norwood, there was a huge furore in the neighbourhood as the Asian family down the road were having an old friend, Sean Connery, to visit. Apparently, the dad used to be a chef in the West End and served all the stars in the sixties. Much excitement as James Bond was massive at that time. Grandpa came up with a reason to go round there at the given time: to return a ladder or some such. Anyway, some confusion – turns out it was a fellow chef called Sean Connelly and he was more Kenneth Williams than James Bond if you get my drift (think Julian Clary).

Michael was by now struggling and we should have realised something was sadly amiss. Truth is, I simply felt irritation and flashes of anger. From where I was sitting, Michael had everything – a flat, a girlfriend, his artwork every day, a nice city to live in, no money concerns, with a constant stream of finance from yours truly.

His reluctance to engage in anything – with us or his work – with any degree of enthusiasm enraged me at times. He was, to my mind, lazy and selfish and thoughtless. I did my best to keep all of that to myself and did so fairly successfully for a while (although Tracey and I would grumble about it together). For now, with Michael, I just kept on joking.

March 2009

Michael,

It's been something of a mixed week. On Monday, your mother left me one of her notes for when I got back from the school run: 'Drier made funny noise. Stopped. Call D & G, we have a policy.' So that was two hours of the morning written off. Yes, the parts are under guarantee; no, the labour isn't covered. Yes, you can get an engineer out but it's approx £100 a call-out.

Inevitably, we didn't have an insurance policy to cover labour (I had forgotten) so I had to sign up to one on the spot to get someone out. I felt I was being ripped off somehow but wasn't sure where. Anyway, the fellow arrived (at

last) on Friday and it turned out a piece of what looked like
kitchen roll had been left in a pocket and worked its way
through to the fan and blocked it. There was a brief flurry
of cashola and it was written down as the starter motor,
which was what your mother had predicted. Everyone
happy.

Talking of your dear mother, she was making various
grunting noises on Tuesday and, eventually giving in as I
could not hear the television properly even turned up to 67,
I asked her what the problem was. She says that she has
some sort of allergy thing and cannot get her breath at
times and that it could be serious. I was, of course, sympathetic and told her to go to the doctors (who are utterly
useless and you usually get some stand-in who cannot
speak English in about three weeks' time). I'm not sure
what my response should have been but I seemed to be on
your mother's blacklist for a good two days.

Anyway, come Friday and your mother announces first
thing that she has now lost her sense of smell. (Something of
an advantage in our house.) None of us quite knew what to
say as your mother said it with a sense of triumph in her
voice (as in 'I told you I was dying') and that's always a tricky
one to handle. We mumbled various contradictory words of
encouragement – I think Adam said, 'Congratulations' – and
off she went, clearly put out with us all.

I do not think her day improved much. They had to make,
as part of one of these endless 'living history' things they do

at school, 'Tudor Gingerbread'. This is a non-cooked (think health and safety) sweetbread made of breadcrumbs and honey, etc., and rolled into a mass and cut into squares. So far, so good – they then had to add red colouring (did they have that in the 1500s?) to about half of the squares so that they could create a sort of chessboard effect. The red squares, according to one ghastly child, apparently looked like raw meat and that set some of the children off. One then shouted out he could SMELL THE GUTS (your mother couldn't, of course) and that triggered a round of gagging and retching. Your mother came home with a headache. So that, by and large, has been this week.

Love

Dad

x

I should say that my dear wife appears here – and elsewhere at regular intervals, no doubt – as something resembling the unseen Mrs Mainwaring in the *Dad's Army* TV series: something of a harridan with an extremely large backside of whom Captain Mainwaring lives in fear and trepidation. I must add a disclaimer that any resemblance to a real person, living or dead, is purely coincidental.

Through the commentary, I talk mostly of me and Michael but, of course, also of 'we', Tracey and me (with, occasionally, 'we' being the family of Tracey, me, Sophie and Adam).

Tracey and I come from similar backgrounds and childhood experiences and we have been together for many years. In some ways, we are much the same – how we view life, how we raise our children and, for good and bad, how we approached Michael during these difficult days. We always meant well, did our best, but didn't often know what the best thing to do was, to rush in or to hold back, watch and wait. Some things we got right, others we got wrong.

In other ways, we are quite different. I am quick to emotion, the instant response of shouting and walking away. I can be moved easily, even to tears, by praise and kind words (I'm much better with nasty emails and trolls, which I ignore, and death threats which I handle with grace and aplomb). All of this, of course, is easier to hide when everything and everyone is kept at arm's length behind one-sided letters, emails and texts. Tracey is steadier and more thoughtful, more likely to give a measured response. The phrase 'Told you so' or its variant 'Told you not to' applies to me as often as it does not, but rarely to Tracey.

Tracey and Michael are alike, calm, placid, easy to get along with, likeable. Sophie and I are much more combustible. Adam leans more towards Michael and Tracey than to Sophie and me. As a family, we tend to keep things buttoned-up but reveal more of ourselves in our sentimentality, keeping letters, cards and mementoes almost for life. Our home is filled with everything from Michael's first school blazer, through each bicycle every child ever had, to childhood videos, games and trinkets and even camping and ski gear they once used. We live in a six-bedroom house by the sea, which sounds grand to some until they realise most of the bedrooms, the loft and the whole of the garage are packed wall to wall, front to back, with all of this beloved junk.

March 2009

Michael,

How is life? Your mother tells me that you are doing cartoons – please don't work too hard. Are we talking cartoons like Disney films or cartoons like Giles? Your mother does not seem to know. I imagine it would be hard to earn much of a living from either: working at a Disney-type studio would be a cut-throat affair I'd imagine – lots of thrusting young executives in shiny suits – and drawing cartoons is not well-paid unless you're a big name like Charles M. Schulz.

Talking of your mother, I got a text whilst doing the school run, 'gerbil dead' (we never know which one is which or what they are called). Great, something to keep me busy when I get home – trying to find a spot in the flowerbeds that doesn't have a dead pet's skeleton in it already and burying the corpse deep enough so that Bernard doesn't dig it up when he goes out to do his business.

Of course, I had expected to find the dead gerbil on the side maybe wrapped in a tea towel with the live one still in the cage. But no – your mother had been 'in a rush' and so the live one was in the cage and the dead one was lying next to it. I'm not sure if the live one was doing the last rites or about to tuck in but I shooed it away and fished out the dead one. Anyway, that's now buried in the garden with a huge stone on top of it. Bernard seemed to be in a state of high excitement (think bloodlust frenzy) as I did the honours, darting in front of me trying to get it dug up before I'd even filled in the hole properly.

We were going to leave this one on its own to try and break the endless first death-replace, second death-replace, first replacement death-replace, second replacement death-replace cycle that we have with both the gerbils and the guinea pigs. But we cracked and got a looky-likey-'Lighty' replacement. I think we will still have these pets the day we die, probably 'Lighty 64' and 'Darky 65'.

Not much else happening. Sophie seems to be giving some thought as to universities and, from what I can make out, the list is, in no particular order, Birmingham, Bristol, Exeter, Durham, York and the University of East Anglia (there is one other I cannot recall). I think UEA may be the one as it is closest so she would not need to rent a place and Lee may be able to get into that too (I think the others, especially Durham, are more upmarket). I said, 'I would be happy to pay for you to go far away,' but your mother thinks I said it with too much enthusiasm and that Sophie was offended. I will keep you posted – I imagine one or other of us will have to do various trips with her at some stage. Your mother annoys Sophie more but I am more embarrassing; a tough choice.

Adam has had some sort of fashionable haircut; it looks as though someone has used a lopsided bowl to do it. It may grow out by the time you see it but, if not, try to say something encouraging. Your mother alleges I said, 'Christ, what were you thinking?' when I first saw it although I do not recall saying that. If I did, it may have been some sort of involuntary reaction. Like myself, I do not think Adam has the face for fashion. He seems to be quite sanguine about it and has the ability, which will prove useful in his life, I'm sure, to laugh at himself. We laughed too (or at least I did) and he took it in good spirits (although it may be that he did not know what I was laughing about).

All for now but do let us know if you are discovered as a cartoon genius. We live in hope that one of our children will drag us out of the mire; we would prefer it to be you than Adam as we will be dragged out that much sooner.

Love

Dad

x

Did any of us still at home – me, Tracey, Sophie and Adam – realise what was happening to Michael? I don't believe we did, not now anyway. Tracey and I never talked then of any great concerns. There was some irritation, for sure. And a dash of anger at times. But we saw much of it as being part of growing up, moving away, finding your feet and all of that. We felt all of our children should make their own mistakes and that they wouldn't stray too far from the straight and narrow because we were all good and nice people.

Neither Sophie nor Adam, still very young admittedly, indicated that they saw anything out of the ordinary or odd. There were no stories that Michael, our quiet and reserved boy, was shouting and screaming, crying, swearing profusely or showing any signs of peculiarity (no more than usual anyway). They were still texting and emailing and all seemed well. If Sophie had suspected anything amiss, she would have told Tracey for sure. Adam too. Tracey and I chewed things over between us but did not share our thoughts and feelings with our two younger children. We wanted them to have warm, happy, Enid Blyton childhoods.

29 March 2009

Hello Michael,

It seems to have been ages since we saw you – are you both well? We should do something soon. We are off to Finlake – me, your mother, Adam – for Easter and Sophie will be here with Bernard (and, no doubt, Lee and a crate of beer). Maybe we could do something when we get back?

Sophie is getting together a schedule of visits to various universities and it seems I am the chosen one when it

comes to ferrying her about. I think it is more to do with
your mother being perceived as having a 'proper job'
whereas I supposedly just sit around all day scribbling bits
and pieces and talking to the postman and the Next deliv-
ery lady as and when they knock.

My money is on UEA because of Lee. Lovely though he is,
drinking aside, I do not think that 'proximity of boyfriend'
should be a key criterion and will try to drop some sort of
observation about that when she is in a good mood (probably ten minutes one afternoon in September). If you can
chip in with a comment as and when, that would be good.
Am I right in thinking Niamh's relatives were or are at
Durham? If so, perhaps you can bring that up and maybe
get them chatting to each other. Sophie should aim high,
higher than UEA anyway – she will be angry with herself
(and all around her) if not.

Your mother seems to have calmed down somewhat. She
went and got various tablets and that seems to have done
the trick. Perhaps, when you next speak, you could ask her
about it all and maybe mention I had been very worried
about it. Phrase that carefully as your mother's stock reply
will be along the lines of 'He's very worried he won't have
his tea on the table at six o'clock', which is a horrible thing
to say.

Maybe you can talk to Adam and see about sorting something out for the Easter holidays – before or after Finlake?
We can come up and see a film maybe and go round the

shops? Or you and Adam can play some computer games whilst we do the rounds? Can you call him?

Love

Dad

x

The main reason that Michael's descent went unnoticed was not that we didn't care, or weren't interested or failed to keep in regular contact with him. We ticked all of those boxes. It was really because ours was a busy and lively household full of robust characters. We all 'got on with it' when it came to working, being ill, getting better, and just doing what needed to be done on a daily basis.

Michael had always been quieter than the rest of us, but when he was at home, he had always seemed to smile and chuckle along with us. He did not seem particularly sensitive or fragile in any way. I assumed – fatal parental mistake, this – that he was much the same as I'd been at that age: reasonably confident, fairly hard-working and with a sense of purpose.

Of the children, Sophie is by far the closest to me in terms of personality and – to her undoubted horror – looks. As I did at that age, she knows what she wants, and goes and gets it. She also has, or had when she was a teenager, a quick temper, as I do, or did – I've learned to control it fairly well over the years (either that or my waning testosterone levels have softened me up).

Sophie's temper left its mark around the house in years gone by, not least a huge dent in the kitchen boiler where her forehead came into contact with it on several occasions in rapid succession. I forget what the matter was at the time – most likely, a top was still in the wash and not yet ready to wear. It would have been something extremely serious like that, for sure.

April 2009

Michael,

I have another 'lively' weekend to report. Sophie was off on some trip so we thought, nice surprise, we – that is me (your mother thinks as 'we', it gets done as 'me') – would redecorate her room for her. We thought she'd be pleased. I could probably stop this letter right now as I don't doubt you are way ahead of me and are already at the *über*-violent, X-certificate ending.

Anyway, Saturday morning I strip off the old wallpaper which is quite a job, and certainly a sweaty one. In the afternoon I wipe down all the walls and paintwork and make sure everything is just as it should be. Grandad Terry would sand all the skirting boards down to the wood and then build them back up again and I suspect your dear mother would like me to do that too but, as I have a life (of sorts), I just sand them lightly to give the paint a bit of grip. It does me just fine. Later, I give the walls a first coat and gloss the picture rails and skirting boards. All done in time for the usual Chinese and everything looking good. (What could possibly go wrong?)

Sunday morning and the back of the door gets a coat of gloss (I had 'forgotten' to do this on Saturday as I thought no one ever sees it as it has Sophie's stuff on a hook on it – I had overlooked your mother, of course). I then dib-dab in the picture rails and the skirting boards where I've missed bits on the Saturday night (it looked like a blind man had had a go at it in places) and try to get the paint out of the edges of the carpet from the day before (some gentle trimming with the nail scissors needed here). Pause for lunch. All looking good. Sophie will be pleased.

Sunday afternoon, and the walls get a second coat between two and four as it gives them two hours to dry before Sophie has to be collected at six. Your dear mother will do this whilst I move all the furniture back in place, and generally get it looking tickety-boo, other than hooks and posters, etc., which will go back up later. It is all just perfect and we are looking forward to seeing the surprise and delight on Sophie's face when she opens the door to see the whole room magically transformed.

It is at this point that I decide to 'walk' the three-door Homebase wardrobe from one side of the room to the other for a better effect when she opens the door. About halfway across I realise why we have never done more than just pull it out to hoover behind it before – in short, it wobbles and tips more than the Leaning Tower of Pisa.

So I can go back or forward or just leave it there in the middle. Thinking quickly, I decide it would be best if I emptied the wardrobe of its contents (I had removed just enough for me to be able to move it but not so many clothes that I would have to spend ages putting everything back). I then try to move it forward (in for a penny, in for a pound) and discover what happens when there are no clothes in it to hold it steady: one end of it seems to stick in the carpet, and leans forward sharply at an impossible angle. I stand it up, it slumps. The only way I can keep it upright is by ramming the whole thing against a wall. Only problem is, to get the wonky end against a wall, the wardrobe will have to face inwards.

Fortunately, only one third of the three-part wardrobe is actually broken beyond repair and I decide – I am now in a dreadful sweat – that if I can remove that, we can present it as a two-piece wardrobe, which 'certainly looks a lot nicer and gives you much more room' (carefully rehearsed). Unfortunately, removing the third bit (shelves mostly) seems to cause the rest of the wardrobe to give way so, to cut a very long story short, I am now sweating and blood-ied, and I broke it all up and threw it piece by piece out of the window onto the front lawn (I was not 'in a temper' as has since been claimed although I admit I may have given that appearance – I have that sort of face). I arrange the wardrobe's contents neatly in six or seven piles roughly where the wardrobe would have been, give or take, and shut the bedroom door.

Sophie comes home and opens the door and you have, near enough, the ending you imagined at the beginning.

Suffice to say, 'surprise', 'delight' and 'magical transformation' did not feature too highly. In fact, they did not feature at all.

Love

Dad

x

Sophie has always been seen by everyone in the outside world as a caring person who would do anything for anyone. I have lost count of the times someone or other has been saying how lovely such and such a girl was, nice to everyone, always helpful, and have had to ask who they were talking about, then do a double-take when they said Sophie.

Looking back at Sophie's teenage years of high drama and drunken slobbery – no different from many teenagers, I suspect – I have to say I see little comparison with the adult Sophie of more recent times.

Even then, though, she was a kind girl at heart. There were nights when she would babysit Adam so Tracey and I could go out. Admittedly, these evenings would often end with frantic texts: *Burglar downstairs!!! What do I do?*; *See if he has time to hoover the lounge?* But the kindness was there underneath it all. There were bunches of flowers and homemade Key lime pies and other little touches now and then too.

17 May 2009

Dear Michael,

Not a lot to report.

Your mother has been shopping for what she calls 'in-between' shoes – I tried not to get drawn into a conversation as I sensed it could prove expensive. From what I can gather, 'in-between' shoes are shoes that are not quite suitable for spring and not quite right for summer; hence, something in between. She worked her way through several pairs in different shops, each time exclaiming that she could get the right one on but not the left. I referred to it as her 'Frankenstein foot', which may seem foolish at first glance as it commits me to two days in the doghouse. Had I expressed interest in in-between fashions, I would have been committed to further outlay, shoes, coats, etc., not just for summer, autumn, winter and spring, but all the in-between seasons as well. In the long-run, I am better off – short-term pain, long-term gain.

Sophie has, not for the first time, blocked ears and this has led to the screaming ab-dabs. Again, not for the first time, I gave in to constant pressure and, against my better judgement and wishes, I drove her to Ipswich A & E. I always feel intensely foolish on such occasions as we sit there amongst old dears with bruised faces, children with broken limbs and assorted teenagers with spikes sticking out of their heads and I have to whisper to a nurse, 'She has a painful ear.'

I always try to make out it is something serious and she has some sort of brain injury, and off she goes, her face contorted with pain, only to return three minutes later having been told to apply olive oil twice a day for the next two weeks. I have lost count of the number of times we have gone through this rigmarole over the years. The only pleasure I got from it this time is that Sophie announced she cannot hear out of either ear so I now speak in a deliberately low voice to annoy her.

Adam woke up earlier in the week screaming – apparently. We all slept through. He tentatively raised it the next morning, 'Did anyone hear . . . ?' He'd dreamed someone was killing him. We'd never have noticed. Once I am asleep, nothing can rouse me. Just after you were born, we slept through that hurricane. Your mother allegedly shook me awake shouting the roof was coming off and I rallied a little to be polite and then went back down. The next morning, the road outside looked like a war zone – all news to me.

It's all very quiet and peaceful here.

Love

Dad

x

If someone had asked me in, say, 2007 which of our three children might possibly go a little wonky, I'd have probably put a fiver, if pressed, on Adam. He is our third child, eleven years younger than

Michael and seven years younger than Sophie. Of course Sophie has told him at certain moments of high emotion (there have been many) that he was an accident – hardly something that is likely to be a confidence-booster to anyone of any age despite our assurances that this was not the case.

Naturally enough, Sophie never considered the possibility that we might have tried for a fourth child (which we did for a long and soul-destroying two years). All she saw was a seven-year gap so, *voilà*, Adam must have been an accident.

At this time, with none of us aware of Michael's woes, Adam was fine. He always seemed happy with the jokes and teasing that are, we think, a natural part of a warm, loving family at ease with each other. He has quite a dry wit himself. But growing up with an older brother who had what turned out to be myriad mental health issues cannot have been easy. In many ways his childhood, certainly his teenage years, unfolded under a dark cloud. And yet, of all of them, 'Big Div', as we now know him, has probably turned out to be the most normal of the three. So much for logic.

June 2009

Dear Michael,

More dramas to report (naturally). It's been the best part of two years now since Sophie heard from Megan. I thought that, like your mother's friendship with Kathy, this one had died a well-deserved death. But no, I – I! – received a text from Megan the other day saying she had passed her driving test and was wondering if Sophie would like to go for a drive with her in her car. She'd been texting Sophie who had not replied. Of course, having always had a soft spot for Megan, I passed it on and, hey presto, there seems to be some sort of line of communication going again. (It won't last, they're chalk and cheese.)

All well and good but then your dear mother has to stick her oar in (for a change). Your mother, seeing an opportunity to get someone to go with her to see *Mamma Mia* in Christchurch Park, then texted Kathy to suggest they all went to it. Kathy, thank goodness, waited four days to reply and then came up with some half-baked nonsense about a family barbecue that night. Your mother was not best pleased as she has been ignoring Kathy for some fifteen months now and only asked her as she had run out of friends for *Mamma Mia*.

How have your courses been going? I assume you have had some sort of tests or what have you and grades? I know you enjoy where you go and all of that but it is possibly not the most prestigious of 'halls of learning' so I think you need to come out with the highest possible grade you can. Sophie has been telling us that a first from, say, UEA is not the same as one from Oxford or Cambridge in the way that A level art is A level art wherever you do it so please do the best you can. This is all costing quite a lot of money one way or the other and you do want to come out with something that will actually be useful. (An embossed certificate with a wax seal framed and mounted on the wall is nice but it is not actually useful; it does not pay the bills.)

I suppose much of it – your art at least, Niamh's medieval stuff is a little different – has more to do with talent than an ability to memorise and regurgitate facts in endless essays. As such, your grade will give you some idea of whether you can make a living from it. Do you have to draw or create things in an exam setting? I hope you do not suffer from nerves. Many years ago, when doing O levels (olden-days GCSEs), I had a friend called David Marsh who had some sort of panic attack whilst doing O level art and drew a cow's legs with a ruler. Incredibly, he still passed.

I would suggest that you really need to be getting a top grade to set off the fact that the Norwich School of Colouring In the Corners is not on the *Sunday Times* Top Universities List (or, truth be told, the *Daily Star*'s). A chap I do some work with – David Bird – said that he got a 'drinker's degree', whatever that is. (I laughed and nodded wisely as if I knew what he was talking about.) Whatever a drinker's degree is – the lowest you can get away with, I guess – I don't think it is very useful to anyone. Think on.

Your dear mother tells me you and Niamh have now become 'proper vegetarians' (whatever that means, is it vegan?). What's that all about? Given the way you used to whoosh down cheeseburgers, I find that a surprising turn of events. Are you short of money? I do not particularly want to up your allowance as things are a little tight this end – but I can do (a little bit) if needs be (at least for the summer if you have spent it all). You must eat properly, and that means some red meat from time to time. You cannot live on beans and pasta and lentils and stuff like that. I do hope it is not to do with this diet business and looking good. You have to be careful not to go too far. The Maitland family are not naturally sleek – we are built like Ladas not Lamborghinis. Think on it please.

Love

Your Poor Father

xx

We return to Michael as he comes to the end of his second year at university and my apparently light-hearted comments that were really a thinly veiled mix of the usual repressed anxiety and anger. I was of the view that Michael was not working particularly hard and that their courses, interesting though they might be, would not be of much use to anyone in the 'real world' (Niamh, so far as I can see, has never really used her Henry VI bag-weaving degree to this day). I did now see my life stretching out with me effectively having to pay for everything for everyone until the day I died, with some debts paid off, at the age of 123.

The eating and the whole vegetarian stance – to be followed, first, by going vegan and then gluten-free in due course – was becoming more of an issue. When Michael was younger, he would wolf down sausages and other great lumps of mashed-up animal without a second thought. Now it became trickier to eat out: we had a 'fussy eater'.

I am not an expert on mental health or anything else for that matter – you'll find little common sense in any of these pages let alone good, solid advice about anything at all (even by luck rather than judgement) – but there is a sense that Michael was now simply putting up obstacles, devising more and more reasons not to eat.

'I cannot eat meat on principle'; 'I am now a vegan, so I cannot eat any of that'; 'It has to be dairy-free'; 'It has to be gluten-free.' By the time he had erected all of these many barriers, there seemed little left to eat but a range of vegetables.

12 July 2009

Dear Michael,

We've just got back from a day out with Granny at Hever Castle – again. (I'm not sure why we seem to go there all the time. I think because it is about halfway and ticks all the boxes: a stately home for Granny and your mother, a maze for Adam and a nice place to eat for me – and home-made stuff too, and not 'homemade' like your mother's I might add.)

We had a nice time as always other than I've noticed that these 'yah, Tristram' parents seem to constantly film their

children these days and invariably get in the way of everyone else who is just being normal. They don't go round the
maze as we do: they film their children going round the
maze and provide a running commentary on how little
Theodore or Pandora is doing. The poor children almost
have to act out a script. ('Do it again, Bethesda, and look
more surprised!') Can they not just have fun themselves?
Why do they always feel they have to film everything?

You and Sophie would just go out and step in dog mess – I
would not have wanted to film that. I am always tempted to
stand close to these pompous 'perfect' parents and do what
your mother calls my 'cor blimey' voice, which apparently I
use when talking to workmen and dockers. It's tempting to
drop one or two expletives in but then I think it would be a
horrible thing to do when the children hear it played back
(but I still imagine doing it for the parents' benefit).

Granny asked after you (perhaps you and Niamh could
come down with us at some stage?). We are thinking of
going to Chartwell with Granny in September, round about
my birthday. Winston Churchill's place in Kent? It's not too
far. We've been trying to find somewhere different to go
other than Hever Castle and the caves and that seems to
tick the boxes. It has lots of things to look at and read –
your mother will spend hours and hours there, no doubt.

Are you getting ready for Spain? I have been doing twice
the usual amount of work to get everything lined up. I
think there is talk of a get-together soon, including Lee,

just to show you the place and the villa on the internet – 'the interweb' to your poor deluded mother – and to talk through timings, etc. Lee has not been on a plane before so we are talking about planes being very safe but also regaling him with stories of plane crashes. There was a very famous one where a plane crashed in the Andes and the survivors had to eat each other. I've been nominated as first in the pot. Talk to your dear mother about it (the get-together, not the feast) and we can maybe set something up for next week or the week after.

Love

Dad

x

PS Your mother has seen a car with a sticker in the back window that reads, 'My Next Husband Will Be Normal'. She said she wanted one. I thought she was going to wait by the car and ask the woman where she got it, no doubt comparing husbands' funny ways. Fortunately, she needed to go to the toilet – an age thing – but has since been telling everyone about it to the point of irritation. I suppose it will become the equivalent over time of my joke, 'My first wife and I married at Gretna Green.'

Some families have a strong support network of grannies and grandads, uncles, aunts and cousins. For us, we were always simply five and there was never the wider family group who might have stepped in, or had a quiet word, or helped to put matters right before everything spiralled downwards and out of control.

In my eyes, my father was a ghastly excuse of a human being who treated my mother shamefully. I left the house when I was eighteen and never saw him or any of that side of the family again. My mother had a mother and father, Nan and Grandpa. I loved Nan and Grandpa (although he was quite crusty on the outside, he was soft within, blowing his nose repeatedly through every episode of *This Is Your Life* to disguise his tears). By 2009, my mother, Michael's granny, was the only family member left on my side.

As for Tracey, her father died suddenly when she was eleven and her mother struggled to cope with that. Tracey left home, with me, when she was seventeen and was not reconciled with her mother for more than twenty years. She has a brother and they are civil to each other. That's a story in itself but for now, suffice to say, there was no extended family support network there – although we were, by 2009, on speaking terms, and comfortable, with Michael's grandma.

Michael had not had the warm relationship with his grandparents that I'd had with Nan and Grandpa: he saw his granny, my mother, a few times a year and later, from when he was fifteen, his grandma too. The closeness I had experienced with my grandparents was missing. It was no one's fault, just that everyone was 100 to 150 miles apart. By 2009, though, he didn't really see them any more, although they sent birthday and Christmas cards and gifts, and he sometimes posted a card or thank-you note to them. It had all drifted away.

Dear Michael,

It's not been the best of weeks – I shall be pleased to get to Spain (are you coming over next Sunday? Do confirm please).

I went to the dentist – it was the usual gauntlet of shame. More fillings needed; refilling fillings really. No, I could not see the hygienist – my teeth are in such a state that scraping and flossing could cause havoc. But I can see some dental assistant who'll show me how to brush my teeth properly. The shame of it. Will she then give me a Tufty Squirrel sticker?

Another guinea pig has died. I'm not sure which one it actually is but don't like to ask in case I am seen as a thoughtless father. Then again, no one else seems to be referring to it by name either so it may be that none of us knows – I buried it in the garden with a homemade cross; the tomb of the unknown guinea pig.

This whole Mini thing is turning into a complete and utter shambles. We went into the dealership in Ipswich to do the paperwork with a debit card and the rusty banger. We were meant to be getting £2,000 for it from the government towards the new Mini; some slippery scheme to kickstart the car industry. Anyhow, long, long story, the Mini is being purchased in your mother's name and the old banger is in my name; *voilà*, we cannot do the deal with the £2,000 allowance. Your mother was not best pleased.

So, the new Mini that was on order for us is now not going to be ours and they are going to have to sell it off their forecourt. We have now ordered another one in my name so that the rusty wreck can be used for £2,000 towards the cost. It's going to be another six weeks before we can get the new Mini, your mother will continue to drive the Picasso that I was going to have and I will continue to drive the old heap. It turns heads at Ipswich School amongst the Mercs and Jags. I feel I should wear pyjamas and a dressing gown to suggest I'm an eccentric but Adam says no, I should be who I am (pause for suspected thought . . . a complete loser).

Do let us know about next weekend – and can you sit next to Lee please and chat to him a bit so he feels at ease with you and Niamh? I know he seems quite confident but your mother, who has made a study of such things, says he may be a little shy and nervous underneath.

Love

Dad

x

Incredibly, or so it seems now we know what Michael was going through at this time, Michael and Niamh actually went on holiday with us, along with Sophie's boyfriend Lee, in August 2009 and all seemed well. It was to be something of a last hurrah for us in terms of holidaying as a family – and, I guess, a last hurrah for us as a happy family as well.

We rented a villa up in the hills of Palamos in Spain and alternated days at the beach with visits further afield, to waterparks and, most memorably, to Barcelona where, in a brand-new hired Mercedes and a far-too-tight underground car park – you're ahead of me – I managed to rip one side to shreds.

More seriously, I have the 2009 holiday photos in front of me now and, comparing them with those from 2007, I can see that Michael is well beyond the 'slim' stage and is now out-and-out thin. His powers of deception must have been considerable (or we were blindly stupid) because even then we simply did not see what was staring us in the face: the long-sleeved T-shirts on the beach; not going for a swim; the clues were all there.

At this time, when Michael and Niamh seemed cheerful and relaxed with each other and all seemed well enough to us, Michael was actually highly stressed and anxious about life generally; my regular jibes about getting 'a proper job' probably didn't help.

And then, wonderfully and marvellously, completely out of the blue, help came from an unexpected quarter. The father of one of Michael's oldest friends called. He actually came round and knocked on the front door of our home. What a brave and wonderful thing to do. What a lovely, decent human being, to step forward when so many others must have looked the other way. He gave us the perfect opportunity to turn things around and to save Michael from what was, frankly, almost certain death. Did we take it? Did we heck.

September 2009

Michael,

I really do not know what to write. I used to write to my
nan once a week on a Sunday to tell her all my news. I
wanted to do the same with you whilst you were away to
make you feel part of things at home. I don't know if I can
do it any more.

Alex Rossi's dad came round whilst me and Adam were at
the football and he talked to Mum.

Alex's dad says you are not well and that we have to do
something about it now – or you will die. How can I even
write that word?

He says you are very thin and that, in the summer, when
you saw Alex, you could not play football any more as your
muscles had wasted away.

We know you are thin but just thought this was how you
wanted to look, with your hair and everything. Tell us it's
not so.

I do not know what to think or say to you. This is the
hardest letter I have ever written; I have started it three
times and torn them up. I don't know what to write to you.
Please call your mum when you get this and tell us what's
going on.

Love
Dad
xxx

Michael had known Alex for about fifteen years. They first met at school when they were about six. Michael went round to Alex's regularly for years but his parents split up and I guess it must have been some time since Alex's dad had seen him. He saw the stark deterioration that had been a slow, gradual process to us.

He was blunt: they'd played football and Michael did not have the strength to run (until he'd gone to Norwich, he'd played Sunday League football once or twice a week and had won a couple of awards). If we did not do something about it now – right now – Michael would die. That was how blunt he was. He gave us our chance. We simply did not take it.

Tracey told me what had been said and there was a sense of realisation between us, a moment when things that had seemed odd fell into place. Yet we did not really take it in, the utter seriousness of it. He was 'thin', 'needed to eat more'; it was a bad situation, even very bad, but it could be turned round with some effort. The idea of death, at this point, seemed so extreme, so unlikely, that it was just impossible to contemplate.

So, we mulled it over between ourselves, umming and aahing, not knowing what to do or say – this was a situation so far removed from our comfort zone, our laissez-faire style of parenting, that we really had no idea how to handle it. We dithered. We stalled. We were not sure.

Tracey talked to Michael on the phone, as she did regularly. I recall a meeting later with Michael and Niamh, her usual breezy manner a little more serious this time but still positive and upbeat. We shuffled around the subject, agreed with the reassurances that Michael had lost some weight but this was all part of growing up and people did change as they got older and it was nothing much to worry about. We let it all slip away.

Looking back, perhaps we should have gone in hard and fast, and tried to have him sectioned straight away. As we ranged over all of the options – from 'wait and see' to 'get professional help' – we considered it. But we saw things spiralling out of control, Michael in a strait-jacket with electric shock therapy, them and us, and shades of Orwell's 1984. So, wait and see, give him a chance to sort things out for himself. That was what we decided to do.

In a way and despite all of the circumstantial evidence that was building up, I think we didn't want to believe it and needed Michael to tell us it was not so. That was exactly what he did and we went along with it. The sad fact is that many people with mental illness, and I think anorexics especially, will do anything and everything to cover their tracks. They lie. They cheat. They steal. They are, after all, not themselves (or not as we wish them to be) and are not 'thinking properly'. They do whatever they need to do to disguise the fact that they are wasting away by not eating. And the ignorance or stupidity of those around them allows them to do just that for so long that, eventually, they die.

October 2009

Dear Michael,

Your dear mother tells me you are basically well and that this whole thinness thing is all part of a 'thin white duke' persona. I'm not hugely reassured that you are following David Bowie's lifestyle. He had a serious drug habit for many years. I recall an interview in which he said he lived on red peppers, cocaine and milk. Hardly a balanced diet. He also sang a song about a laughing gnome, which was downright peculiar.

I thought it was big-hearted of Alex's dad to come round and say what he did. It took courage and, mistaken or not, it was done with the best of intentions for sure. I imagine something got lost in translation between Alex, his dad, your dear mother and then me. Heaven knows, we are easily confused. It was just such a shock – excuse my over-reaction. These 'looks' of yours are all well and good but you have to be careful not to go too far with them.

Back in the eighties, there was a pop group called Ultravox. Their lead singer Midge Ure was very popular – Band Aid? Anyway, he had a pencil-thin moustache and I decided to grow one too. Only problem, my hair was dark brown and my moustache came out a sort of dirty blond. Not a good look, so I dyed it with one of these Superdrug kits. Quite a decent match except when the sunlight hit it and it turned purple. So, when talking to people outdoors, I'd suddenly notice they were no longer looking at my eyes but my upper lip. I know what it must be like to be a girl with a large chest.

Your dear mother also tells me that (a) you have no secrets from us, and (b) you are not gay; (a) that's good to hear, and (b) I never thought you were. Odd, yes. Gay, no. I have always been able to spot a gay or lesbian almost instantly. There was a man who used to live next door to us who wore very tight shorts and would spend hours in the back garden on a child's swing. I spotted him early on. Women can be trickier but the hands are often a giveaway. Remember Huge Janet? Great big spade hands – always a tell-tale sign.

I would not be bothered if you were gay, quite honestly (although I imagine Niamh may have something to say about it). The onus on delivering grandchildren – not yet, please – would then fall to Sophie and, I assume, Lee, and that would be a concern. He is a nice-looking boy but lazes about much of the time to the point of being comatose, and he drinks like a fish; not a terrific combination when it comes to passing on genes.

Please do humour us and try to keep an eye on your weight (your dear mother will worry and I will have to bear the consequences). I have found that these BMI (Body Mass Index) charts that you can get online are rather useful as it takes your height into account. They offer a range of weights according to whether you are big-boned or not. If I put an extra two inches on my height – I am not sure if I am six foot or six two – I am borderline obese and can live with that. Your mother who is short but not fat has suffered from losing two inches in recent years so she does not use these charts any more.

We are looking forward to seeing you again for another meal. Do let us have your birthday list just as soon as you can and book somewhere nice to eat in Norwich. Don't forget Adam's birthday – talk to your mad sister but Wimpy Kid and Batman are popular right now; figurines etc.? If you are short of money – don't tell me – you can draw a picture for him and maybe frame it?

Love

Dad

x

So there we have it, an unequivocal denial from Michael that anything was wrong. The 'I'm fine' line was a constant message for some time to come, despite the evidence before us as Michael became thinner and thinner still.

We, too, were in denial. We knew now that Michael wasn't 'quite right' but didn't see it in the life and death terms that his friend's father had spelled out to us.

Michael could never die. How could he?

And how could anything bad ever happen to us, our jolly, loving family?

It was unthinkable.

Someone we knew, not so very long ago, told us that they thought we were the perfect family – all doing well, getting on together, laughing and joking – and that was how we saw ourselves.

We could face difficult issues – we'd seen plenty in our wider families in the past, including teenage death, suicide and even a gruesome demise by rotten teeth. But we didn't think anything bad could ever happen to any of us five. We were immune.

So we smiled and laughed, and carried on pretty much as we were, and assumed Michael was doing the same. Fact is, as we smiled and laughed, Michael was moving slowly but surely towards his own demise.

18 October 2009

Dear Michael,

I know we are not to worry, and all is well and hunky-dory, and we are overreacting (as per) but I really do think you are looking terribly thin. I had not realised before. I did not want to say anything at your birthday meal or at Adam's Chinese, but you really do not look like a Maitland at all (three cheers, you might well say, given that we are 'the fatty family').

I have not always been the bloated wreck you see before you. When I was your age, I was six foot and thirteen stone. I had a round face and solid arms and legs (my legs are quite short compared to my body, but that's another story). All in all, I was meaty. Prime beef, you might say. You are more chicken leg. Your face has almost no flesh on it and your arms and legs are like sticks. Think *A Nightmare Before Christmas* and an L. S. Lowry painting.

I am your father – if I do not say these horrible nasty things to you, no one else will. You need to sort this out.

Putting on weight is a simple business; God knows it's an upward curve for me all the time. Weigh yourself as of today. Then eat three square meals a day. Do a little exercise but not too much; a walk or a swim every (other) day. Eat some meat each day. A little bit of chocolate. Have a doughnut now and then. Weigh yourself once a week and then see how much you have put on in, say, a month. Aim for a couple of pounds a month. Simple.

I have not said anything to your dear mother. She will only worry and we will have to discuss this over and over again. (Maternal Motto: 'Why say something once when you can say it many, many times?') I think you have simply taken your 'look' too far; you don't want to be the thin white duke. Or, on the other hand, Buster Bloodvessel (Google 'Bad Manners'). Something in between? Your mother likes that man from the Pet Shop Boys (the one who sings, not the one who prances about in the background). Why not look like him?

Anyway, let us say no more on this subject. It reminds me of the time I had to come and get you from school and take you to hospital [Michael had suffered a 'down below' injury during some horseplay]. Embarrassing all round really. I do not mind addressing sensitive issues if I have to but I do not wish to dwell unduly on matters. I'd rather 'get on with things'. So get on with this and let's have a proper look at you at Christmas.

Love

Dad

PS We will give you a 'bye' weight-wise when we see you on your mother's birthday. But do please avoid the three jumpers routine – anyone who wears multiple layers of the same clothing is either too skinny or barking mad (or quite possibly both). And don't ask your mother her age – she is forty-five, if you must know.

PPS Your dear mother took to asking me recently, when passing a woman of indeterminate age, 'Does that woman look older or younger than me?' I'd say, 'Younger,' simply to annoy her. 'Much younger,' if I was feeling particularly chippy (and my dinner that day was not at risk).

PPPS Your mother then thought she had sussed me out. 'How old do you think that woman looks?' 'Younger than you', 'Much younger than you', etc. Simple pleasures, really. I take them as and when I can.

I am not what you might call 'a man's man'. I do not have 'mates' with whom I go to pubs and stagger back legless wearing a traffic cone on my head or covering my bare buttocks. I am not very good at banter and I could not chat up a woman even if my life depended on it. I do not smoke or drink: I blow when I should suck and I slump sideways after a pint and a half. I am, as my dear wife would say, 'a bit useless' in that department (and, no doubt, many others).

A 'man-to-man' chat is not something I could have face to face to Michael. I shy away from such matters. No 'facts of life' chats for us. No discussions about what my own mother would have referred to vaguely as 'down there' matters. No serious fatherly advice on love-related issues of a romantic or a physical nature. What 'advice' I do give – telling an anorexic to eat three square meals a day about sums it up – is often unintentionally risible.

1 November 2009

Dear Michael,

Do you and Niamh do fireworks or are you 'too old' these days? There are many things you can never be too old for in my opinion – fireworks, Cadbury Creme eggs, snowballs, dolly mixtures and the *Doctor Who Christmas Annual* (note) come to mind. I have, in recent years, removed 'kicking piles of leaves' from this list as I have noticed that Bernard always makes a beeline for these when he needs to do his business. 'Sticking your head out of train windows' – very popular in my younger days – has gone too after I read a story about someone's head being torn off and lost somewhere along the tracks.

We have found a new fireworks place – it's a pub (name escapes me) over near Woodbridge where you went paintball-ing. They have a small bonfire and you can get a nice pint (half for your mother) and proper burgers and hot dogs (we go back once or twice) before the fireworks at 7.45ish. They last about fifteen minutes – that's plenty – and everyone then clears off. You can pay what you want. Bonus. It's all fairly civilised without too many teenagers pushing and shoving and effing and blinding all the time. We stopped going to Christchurch Park a year or two back after I stumbled over a girl going to the toilet and Adam trod in dog dirt.

Your mother's birthday (before you ask) – I am potless ideas-wise. As you may have heard, last time out, we went round Ipswich one Sunday just prior and your mother carefully pointed at assorted items in Debenhams, Accessorize and H & M. The idea was that I would then go back and buy 'some' (i.e. 'all') of these items for her birthday. Needless to say, I got confused as I think they must have moved stuff around in the ten minutes in between (just my luck). I picked the wrong scarf in Accessorize (right colour, though) and the wrong handbag in Debenhams (which I was duly told was more of a 'manbag', whatever that is).

This year, we went round together, your mother, my debit card and I, and we chose some really nice items, coat, etc., which I have put aside for the big day. I will then fill it out with one or two bits. Books, vouchers and CDs (Take That excepted) always generate black looks and/or dark comments so I am getting some perfume this year (having inspected what is being used at present and checked levels). Perhaps have a talk to Sophie and Adam; Sophie seems quite good at picking clothes for your mother in so far as your mother always seems pleased to receive them and Sophie always seems pleased to wear them.

A painting of the dog, just 'head and shoulders' (do dogs have shoulders?), would be good but I fear your mother would consider that more of a present for me than for her; so maybe file that one away under 'Surprise Presents for Dad'. You will need to have a photo if or when you do this – Marji had a painting done of her dog by a girl who was selling stuff at 'Art on the Prom' in September. Turned out nothing like the dog. Marji ventured the girl had worked from a stock photo off Google. Your mother wondered whether she was not an artist but was simply selling sticky buns on the prom. I suggested the girl may have been blind. Grandpa used to buy art from people with no hands and no feet; very good they were too (although, obviously, they bore no likeness to anything).

Well, we'll leave it there. We will come up to you on birthday night as there is a greater choice of places to eat than here. It's either the Alex or the Wimpy or assorted pubs frequented by grunting dockers round here. Give your mother a call mid-week?

Love

Dad

x

PS By the by, your mother's 'allergies' are back. She will cough at an early stage of meeting up and, if you do not pick up on it, will repeat it until you do. Ask early how she is and we can then crack on with the meal. Otherwise she will only cough all the way through.

And so, just a few weeks after we had been told that unless Michael turned things around immediately he would die, normal service was resumed as if nothing had ever been said. I continued with my stream of nonsense and trivia aimed at making Michael and myself laugh (and not necessarily in that order).

The reality was that Michael now spent much of his time curled up in bed, when he was not cocooned in the cinema, he ate less and less, and did relatively little work at university. Niamh, still a young girl and with no experience of these things, kept everything to herself, protecting and shielding Michael from the world, including us.

Meantime, I just kept on joking. I assumed, in much the same way that I must have imagined Michael would pick up on the facts of life without any input from me, that this turnaround would somehow take place as if by magic with nothing being said or done to encourage it. By now, though, any magic that had once been sprinkled over us all had long since blown away.

November 2009

Hello Michael,

I expect you know all the latest news by now – you probably heard it all from Norwich – but, in case you don't, Sophie and Lee have split up. It all happened on Saturday when your mother had taken Adam to someone or other's party and Sophie and Lee were at home upstairs whilst I had unpacked and was playing with my new leaf sucker and blower in the garden. (It blows brilliantly but sucks at sucking as you have to get it at a certain angle to pick up leaves and only a small number at a time and not wet ones. All a bit rubbish really.)

Anyway, I was in a world of my own (some sort of Doctor Who and the Daleks fight) when Lee rushes by, apologising for all the noise and how it was nice knowing me. Odd, me thinks. I had not heard any noise as I was blowing leaves for the previous twenty minutes but thought I had better go upstairs to make some sort of encouraging comments to Sophie.

The door was shut and she seemed to be doing some sort of whirling thing in there like that girl in *The Exorcist*. I think things were being broken and there were lots of shouts and muttered oaths that you do not expect to hear from a former head girl. So, mindful of previous occasions where I have come off worst when I have tried to be kind (think last geography trip), I slipped back to my sucker-blower thing and carried on until your dear mother returned to enter the eye of the storm.

Bottom line? Lee has gone. A shame, for all of his laddishness and drinking (oft-reported but never witnessed by my good self), he was always polite and friendly to us and your mother had a soft spot for him. Poignantly, there are cheesy pizzas and ranch burgers still stacked in the fridge for him. I imagine Sophie, when she spots them, will take them out and stamp on them.

On the upside, we have also seen the last – please, God – of Megan Robertson. She had reappeared (again) at

half-term. Sophie kept calling her in tears for help on
Saturday night when Lee went off. She said she'd come over
but never did. End of things I think. To be fair, she has
spent the best part of two years trying to rebuild her friendship with Sophie who has blanked her, but then when
Sophie opened up, Megan messed her about . . . again.
Girls, eh? Boys would just have a punch-up and then get on
with things.

That's not all. We – me, your dear mother, Sophie and
Adam – decided to go to the fireworks at the football
ground to cheer ourselves up and, don't you just know, we
are standing there waiting, and the Robertsons, one by one,
turn up. Mark nodded, then went and stood ten yards away
with the boy. Megan walked by, pulling a hood over her
head and turning away (a real knife in the heart, that).

Kathy at least came up to us and said hello. I then said,
'Should we talk about Megan?' Your mother said nothing.
She said nothing. I then said, 'Yes, no?' Your mother stared
at the ground. She then said, 'Obviously not,' and walked
off to the rest of them. We stood there for a minute or two
and then shuffled away into the crowd. If the ground could
have opened up and swallowed me at that moment I would
not have struggled much. Once, we were such good friends
– to think we have come to this . . . a truly horrible ending.

Love

Dad

x

Lee was Sophie's first boyfriend and they were together for three years or so. We liked him – before they went out, he came round and introduced himself in much the same way, in ye olden days, as a man would go to his prospective father-in-law for permission to ask his daughter for her hand in marriage. He got on well with Adam, although he had little or nothing in common with Michael.

Our friendship with the Robertsons, once so close, finally ended at the close of 2009, although it was some time before we got over it. We have not spoken to them since then – again, it is another 'if only' when we look back.

Michael was now isolating himself. He had friends – Alex, Toby, Paul in particular – whom he'd known from early schooldays, but he was not in contact with them. Neither, being so wrapped up in himself and Niamh, did he seem to have any friends at university. As he no longer did karate or football, any friendships there had dwindled and died. He was starting to rely more and more on Niamh to do everything, say what needed to be said, to cover for him. And she did. For ages. And ages. Simply ages.

15 November 2009

Dear Michael,

Not a lot happening here at home other than the usual mayhem and mishaps. Your mother is happy with her work at school. The other day, three boys had a farting contest (you are ahead of me already). Two performed perfectly, one was over-enthusiastic and spent some time being avoided by his classmates. One then dubbed him, not unreasonably, 'Stinky Pants' at which point he had hysterics and had to be led away. Fortunately, at eight, he is responsible for 'sorting himself out', which was a job – no pun intended – that your mother was pleased to avoid.

The dog has fleas. I came down to find Adam asleep on the sofa. It seems there were three or four fleas jumping around in his bed in the night. He says it's the dog. The dog just stares us out. As you can imagine, your mother has pretty much stripped every piece of furniture in the house, sheets, pillows, duvets, cushions, throws, even in rooms where the dog doesn't go. It's like Mr Wu's laundry here.

Sophie was sent up to the vet to get some more flea treatment, different from the one we have been using. Your mother, drawing on her PhD in Veterinary Know-All, has decided that the dog has become immune to what we've been using. Personally, I think the three or four simply jumped ship from the mangy old mutt that gave Bernard the all-over sniff treatment a day or so ago when we were out walking. I kept quiet on that one; otherwise, it would be my fault (obviously). Your mother keeps talking about eggs hatching and looks at the dog as if he were a walking time bomb. Think the Great Plague of London . . . started by Bernard.

Your mother has indicated she wants to have an Indian on her birthday and has commented on the nice little knick-knacks in the antiquey-type shops in the alleyways in

Norwich. I pass this information on more in hope than expectation that you can 'attend to matters'.

We'll get to you for about half seven. Listen for the buzzer this time please (especially if it's raining hard – we do not have time for your mother to go into the 'I must sort my hair' routine).

Love

Dad

PS I dread to ask but feel I should – how are you getting along money-wise? You're a student so things should be tight for you but not so tight that you are at breaking point. Let me know – if you must.

PPS Sophie is back with Lee. Your mother is pleased. The fridge is being restocked with ready-to-heat burgers and all-cheese pizzas. It was just a lovers' tiff (sigh).

We were still getting together for birthday meals, which must have been torture for Michael and, indeed, Niamh. It was a busy time of year with four of us having birthdays in a ten-week period. Off we'd troop, apparently all cheerful, to a range of restaurants, Italian, Chinese, Indian, Mexican. We'd shovel down piles of shared starters, main courses with extras, desserts and coffees and shots galore.

Niamh was their smiling face, lively, bouncy, and interested in what we had to say. In retrospect, it took our eyes away from a sick and weary Michael. It must have been agony for her to sit there, bright-eyed and jolly, knowing that when they got home he would pull away, slide into bed, dragging the covers over himself, locked away in his own little world.

When you have an adult child who has always been quiet and self-contained – now quiet, self-contained and thin – it is not always easy to spot the differences between 'quiet' or 'listless' and 'self-contained' or 'unhappy'. Had this been Sophie, our 'Foggy Foghorn', we'd have seen something was not right immediately. With Michael, who didn't want us to see that anything was wrong, it was so much harder to spot what was happening. A smile now and then and the odd comment here and there were all it took to fool us.

29 November 2009

Dear Michael,

I am, I think you will agree, a Christmas enthusiast – unlike Grandpa, who would put decorations up the day before Christmas Eve and take them down the day after Boxing Day with an emphatic, 'That's that for another year then.' Fun and games, such as they were, most definitely over. However, there are some things that annoy me at this time of year . . .

Christmas from October – Grandpa's five-day Xmas-fest may have been short but I am not a fan of two-month

Christmas festivities, which seem to start before Hallowe'en. A card shop in town had the full works decorations-wise and Christmas tunes playing in the third week of October this year. The idiot on the high road had some sort of lights affair in his front window from before Hallowe'en.

Talking Hallowe'en, we had a queue of assorted ghosts and ghouls this year; opening the front gate and putting a lighted pumpkin in the porch seemed to do the trick. Only thing is, most of the adults who visit, with children I hasten to add, seem to have lived here at some stage or other in their lives. Your mother, being a soft sort, ends up showing them around. I cannot help but think these are would-be burglars 'casing the joint'. Thank goodness we have nothing worth stealing (one full and complete set of all *Doctor Who* DVDs excepted).

As for fireworks night, it should be fireworks month (if not longer). They still seem to start round here just after Hallowe'en and then go on right through to New Year when the boats all sound their horns. The dog does not know whether he is coming or going. He leaves the house all jaunty and cock-a-hoop, trotting along and investigating a range of smells, cracks in fences and assorted piles of stuff. Next there's the whoosh of a firework, a bang, and he's scurrying home head-down.

Anyway, Christmas – I am not keen on this trend for competitive decorations. I accept we will have several Christmas trees and decorations throughout the house but these are for our own joy and delight and no one else's. I'm talking those maniacs – only word for them – who have outdoor lights from top to bottom, life-sized Santas and snowmen in the garden and put them up right at the start of December if not earlier. Some of them try to justify it by nailing a charity tin to the fence and asking for donations to some unspecified charity. They then go whining to the local press when they've only raised 25p and some lowlife has run off with it.

I cannot stand people who do things for show. It's like these smug so-and-sos who wear poppies all the time – 'Look at me caring.' They most probably paid ten pence for them ten years ago and put them away carefully each year to use them again the next. There's a man down the road – man in a suit – who has had a big poppy on the front of his car for at least five years; I think we are meant to be impressed.

Giving to charity should be a private matter. These days, everyone has to make a song and dance about it, sitting in a bowl of jelly, running backwards with your pants on your head, doing a three-legged race through mud, etc. Look at me! Look at me! Look at me! This all started when Princess Diana died – a tragedy, of course (although no one ever seems to mention that she would probably have survived if she'd bothered with something called a seatbelt). Everyone weeping and wailing as if they knew her personally; we went to a dog show at the RSPCA at Martlesham the day after she died and we had to stand and go through some sort of ghastly minute's silence charade to show we all cared. I thought the woman next to me (not your mother) was never going to get her next breath she was sobbing and gasping so much. She deserved a rosette for that performance.

Anyway, after all that, I am writing to ask if you know yet what you are doing for Christmas: are you and Niamh coming to us or to Niamh's folks or half-and-half? You are both welcome here for a few days. If her parents are divorced now or divorcing – we do not like to ask – I suggest you'd best keep out of it. Things can get very strained at Christmas. Years ago, your Step Uncle Peter went to his mother's for Christmas Day dinner and he had some sort of argument with the current husband (number five, I think, maybe six). It started over the husband having a large hair growing out of his nose. It ended up with them rolling around the floor trying to strangle each other. Talk about *EastEnders*. Talk to Niamh and then tell your mother. Sooner not later please.

Love

Dad

PS I am still swimming – thirty to forty-five minutes a day, Monday to Friday – but have had to step back (gingerly) this week as I have caught some sort of horrible verruca. Have you ever had one? My first, really quite bad. Your devoted mother has been assisting with nail files, ice, etc., to no avail. She said I could still swim if I went and bought a 'verruca sock'. I misheard and have been asking for a 'verruca stocking', much to the amusement of the women in the chemist's.

Christmas must surely be the worst time of the year for an anorexic, especially one who is trying to appear as if everything is normal. Michael and Niamh's first Christmas, 2007, was to be spent apart, although the knock on the door at four o'clock on Christmas Day signalled Niamh's (not totally unexpected) arrival. The year 2008 saw them spend Christmas partly with us and partly with her folks. As we approached Christmas 2009, we were not sure what was going to happen.

We'd noticed earlier in the year, when we'd gone to see Ipswich play Chelsea in London, that Michael was becoming increasingly indecisive. He could not do anything without going round and round in himself and back and forth with us. He seemed incapable of making even the simplest decision; whether to book a table for seven thirty or eight, for example.

This was mildly amusing for a while but it soon became frustrating to everyone. Clearly, it was all part of Michael's wider range of issues. He was like a small child, unable to take any decision for himself and wanting others to make them for him.

As we moved into 2010, Niamh started to make more and more decisions on his behalf. It came to a point where, not realising the full significance of this, we felt Michael could do nothing unless he checked with her first. As such, there was a lot of buttoned-up, hard-to-suppress anger from us, much of it directed – wrongly – at Niamh.

December 2009

Michael,

I recall reading somewhere that a life sentence these days is actually eleven years – so, if you wanted to kill someone really badly (a tax inspector, John Barrowman, an idiot who drives in the middle lane at 50 m.p.h.) you could be out by the time you are thirty-four. Not bad, really. I said something of the sort to Adam recently and he thought about it (cogs whirring and clicking slowly into place) and said he wished he had killed one of the Teletubbies when he was five so he could have missed all his schooling, which I thought was quite funny (but don't tell your mother).

I mention all this as I have, as of four days ago, been with your dear mother for thirty years. The Queen has two birthdays – her actual one and an official one (I do not know why or when but it is a fact nonetheless). Similarly, we have two anniversaries – 1 April, when we married at Gretna Green, and 2 December, when we met in downtown New Malden. It can prove expensive.

There are, when it's all boiled down, few things that are truly important in life. Whether you get an A or a B in a particular GCSE, if your car is new or old, whether you have the latest computer console or not, whether you have a thin TV or a fat TV, if you pay a bill today or next week – almost all of it is just detritus.

As Kathy Robertson once said on that holiday from Hell in Orlando, 'When I was young, all I wanted when I grew up was to be married and have children and be happy.' And that, with minor variations for age, gender and sexual orientation, is near enough what it's all about, 'being happy'.

If you are with the right person, your life is enriched and all the ghastly stuff that comes your way – the work you do not want to do, the people you have to be polite to, the rudeness and hassles of modern life, the bills and taxes you have to pay – just passes you by eventually. The right person is always there. I am not sure what I am really trying to say here – possibly something nice about your dear mother. I draw back in the nick of time.

I guess, when all is said and done, it's things like family and birthdays and Christmases and all that stuff that are important and which endure, and most of the rest of it isn't and won't. I suppose the fact that you are thin and peculiar does not really matter – when we look back in twenty years (if I'm not stone cold dead by then), we will just remember the Christmas Eve pantos, the birthday meals at the Alex, the funny things that always seemed to happen to us on holidays and, as your mother would no doubt chip in at this point, 'That time your dad's trunks came off on the waterpark slide at Aqualand and he ended up on Facebook.' Happy times.

Love

Dad

PS Sophie and Lee have now broken up again (and this time we think it may be permanent).

Heaven forbid, I come close – dangerously close – to saying I love my wife and, quite possibly, my children, too, at this point. I wonder whether, had I done so, it might have stopped Michael from going into freefall.

In all honesty, he was already over the edge and falling fast. Perhaps if I had said it when he was five and kept on saying it, and shown it in more demonstrative gestures, things would not have gone the way they did.

Nowadays, older and possibly wiser (or at least a little less stupid), I tend to think we are what we are and that, with minor and often temporary tweaks in our behaviour for the ones we love, is how we will be throughout our lives.

I look around me now at people I know and I think it is relatively easy to see those who are angry or sad, violent or loving, those who are kind and those who are mean-spirited. The tragedy was that I could not see Michael for what he was.

December 2009

Michael,

We really do not mind what you do at Christmas – it's up to you. Come here alone. Go there with Niamh. Both of you come here. Neither of you come here. It's your choice. Just let us know asap please – your mother is starting to twitch about it and, as ever, I am blamed for everything. Apparently, I have been particularly irritating this week . . .

Revels. We tend to share some chocolate at about 10 p.m. I cannot eat toffees (stumps and crowns) so I leave the toffee Revels, with bite marks, in a neat and tidy row on the coffee table in front of her.

Driving. As you know I do not worry too much about gears. Driving round corners, roundabouts and up Bent Hill in fourth gear seems to annoy. There is also what your mother calls my 'whiplash stops', which I do instead of 'progressive braking', whatever that might be.

'Uh?' Apparently, I do not listen to your mother and when she stops talking (not very often, maybe once or twice a week) and there is a silence I suddenly realise I was meant to have replied and so I say, 'Uh?' This infuriates your mother.

I could go on (and on) but let us leave it there and go back to where we started. Christmas – do it as a couple?

Why not come to the Wolsey panto (we have enough tickets) and then spend your Christmas Day with Niamh's folks and your Boxing Day with us (or vice versa)? We are, as they say, 'cool' with whatever way you go. I am, of course, fairly flexible too. We (i.e. your mother) just need to know for the food.

Love

Dad

PS You will need to let us have some lists and some ideas for Niamh, please. I do not mind doing theatre tickets or something at the O2 that you might both like? Talk to your mother – when you call her this week to confirm your Christmas plans – and exchange some thoughts. Please remember Sophie and Adam too. We will do a family present for Lee (subject to what's happening) – probably Jack Daniel's (although, truth be told, I think he drinks anything, only drawing the line at screenwash and WD40).

PPS If you get a chance to talk to Sophie about universities over Christmas, that would be helpful. We think she would be happier and more contented in the long-run at a place like York or Durham rather than UEA where she can be with Lee (subject to if they are on or off at any given time). I do not think UEA is that great from what I have been reading. York is quite prestigious and an easy enough run for a day out or a halfway meet-up.

And so we come to Christmas, when we did not see Michael or Niamh at what we might call 'eating times', and to the end of 2009 when we should have realised Michael was seriously ill.

The fact is, we were told about it. We saw it with our own eyes. All the signs were there. We ignored them and turned the other way. We could not face up to the reality, did not want to engage with it and hoped, against all reason, that it would somehow sort itself out.

The year 2010 loomed, with Michael's and Niamh's degree courses coming to an end. We expected them to get jobs, move into the real world and stand on their own two feet. Again, we were wrong. We were horribly wrong – 2010 was not to be the best of years.

2010

'You Don't Have to Be a Fairy to Carry a Pink Handbag', 'How to Move a Washing Machine with Your Little Finger' and 'Why You Should Eat 65 Grapes with a Plastic Teaspoon in the Next 3 Minutes'. The year started much the same as ever. I was still writing stuff and nonsense for newsletters and magazines while Tracey was still on poo and wee duty with the little ones at the local primary. (To misquote Mr Spock, or whoever it was on *Star Trek*, 'It's life, Jim, but not as we know it.')

Sophie would take her A levels in June – a new A* grade was being introduced and, inevitably, she was now setting her sights on achieving three A*s and going to the best possible university. 'Hurricane Sophie' was coming in the summer but, as per, we did not see it, let alone barricade ourselves in somewhere safe against the onslaught. May God help us and have mercy on our souls.

Adam, subject to a maths and English entrance exam, would move to his senior school. There was a suggestion that we might send a doppelganger in his place to sit the exam but the fact that he'd now been at the lower school for five years made that an unlikely scenario. We thought his best chance was to have some sort of fit on the day itself.

Life for Michael and Niamh was to reach a crisis point in 2010. Michael was no longer getting up, going to university regularly, doing the work he needed to do to get a good degree. He was pretty much hidden away from the world. We saw him less and less. Niamh, as ever, was upbeat, indicating they were job hunting and had plans for when their degrees ended in the summer.

10 January 2010

Dear Michael,

I guess, being fifty next year (groan), it's a little late to start setting New Year resolutions for the first time. If I did, though, I think it would be to 'do something different'. There are times when I feel as though I have been living a personal 'Groundhog Day' for the past twenty-five years. The only difference is that, when I look in the mirror, I now see a grey-haired, saggy-faced old man looking back at me (yes, it's me I'm talking about, not the old bloke over the road come to share my bathroom).

Twenty-five years I've spent sitting in a bedroom day after day, churning out endless articles on subjects I know little or nothing about. I started, when you were born, as a 'baby equipment expert' for *Baby* and *Mother & Baby* magazines writing about the various pros and cons of buggies, breast pumps and baby-walkers I'd never seen, let alone used.

I progressed via car and lifestyle magazines writing about 'green issues' I knew nothing (and cared even less) about. Memorable quote from one editor: 'Iain, do you even know what a catalytic converter is?'

I ended up with newsletters for publishers of varying repute and have spent the last twelve years or so writing articles such as 'Why You Should Make a Hole in a Postcard Big Enough to Fit Your Head Through' and 'How to Transform Your Appearance with Haemorrhoidal Cream'. 'How to Write a Load of Old Cobblers for Money' best sums it all up.

Of course, it's not easy to 'do something different' when you are my age. You end up with a mortgage, bills to pay, incessant taxes and all of the other outgoings that need to be met before you can relax and enjoy yourself (for about three minutes on a Sunday evening before starting the whole process all over again). There are times when I can barely stretch my earnings and overdrafts and robbing Peter to pay Paul to meet everything that needs to be paid on time.

I think what I am trying to say to you as a New Year offering (no money, I'm afraid), and with the benefit of twenty-five years' hindsight, is that you should 'do something different' now before you get set into the train tracks of life. Decide what it is you want to do and go for that before you have to settle into everyday matters.

When I was young, I always imagined myself as a great novelist – a Hemingway or a Steinbeck – but mortgages and taxes and life got in the way. I was always going to do it tomorrow. There was always an absence of time. Talent too. And then tomorrow became yesterday and last week and, finally, a distant memory. So, whatever you are going to do, do it now. Otherwise, you will wake up one morning and it will be too late; your life will almost all be behind you. Mine seems to be.

Love

Dad

PS The electricity company is asking customers if they have swine flu before sending in engineers to service boilers. Pause for thought. When the meter reader/market researcher/taxman/Jehovah's Witness next comes knocking, just lick your lips as if they were rather sticky and say, 'I'm sorry, you can't come in, I have swine flu.' Perfect.

I had, despite my wearied tone, been a successful professional writer of books, articles and, most recently, newsletters for many years. I have never had what anyone might consider to be a normal nine-to-five, man-in-a-suit type job. In my twenties, after several years of unemployment and a failed baby-shop business just behind me, now married, Michael on the way, no job and no money, I somehow blundered my way into working as a lecturer teaching beauty therapists, despite a complete absence of know-how, experience or qualifications. It was a Friday afternoon. They needed someone, anyone, for Monday morning. I spent most lessons in a sweat, one or two pages ahead of the students.

I continued my teaching career, such as it was – colleges, adult education centres and the odd school – on and off for several years while I continued to write about anything and everything that came my way to pay the bills. Eventually, I gave up teaching – I was doing well enough from writing. I had, in later times at least, made a decent enough living from it and many people, looking at what I'd written, my list of publishers and where I'd been published – all over the world – would have considered me to be something of a somebody.

I've churned out thousands of words a day on a range of topics and it's been a good life, really. But now and then, especially during the January blues, it could seem as dull and automatic as putting on that grey suit and working nine-to-five at some office, wasting my life counting beans, ticking boxes and moving pieces of paper from one pile to another, then back again, day after day.

I wanted Michael's life to be vibrant, colourful and free. My grandpa, married with children and a mortgage, had the choice of being a professional musician or getting a monthly wage in a factory. He chose the regular money. My father wanted to be an antiques dealer – he chose to work at the Midland Bank, again for that monthly payment. I had broken free to be a writer – some achievement, really, to earn a living year in, year out from it. I hoped Michael would do the same and go on to be a successful artist, cartoonist, illustrator, film-maker, whatever, anything but a man in a grey suit.

At the start of 2010, I fondly imagined Michael beavering away at his art, pitching it day after day to publications, galleries, film studios, anywhere that might give him some work, much as I had done in the early years, throwing everything I had as hard as I could against the wall to see what would stick, waiting for the call or letter that would offer me a breakthrough for a new book, a new magazine or something else that was different and another challenge for me. Michael was, I still assumed, like me, and was already up and out there, attacking the world as hard as he could. The reality, of course, was that Michael had that duvet pulled up and over his head to keep the outside world as far away as possible.

17 January 2010

Dear Michael,

There are certain years which, with the benefit of hindsight, are 'historic' ones in the Maitland family – I am not talking obvious ones like 1987, 1992 and 1998. I am talking life-changing years.

The last one was 2007 – your dear mother stopped working for the photography studio after eighteen years. She then started working at the primary; something she should have done years ago. Loves it. Hard work, though. I could not be 'on show' all the time like that without shouting at someone.

We broke off contact with Hilde who said some terrible things about your dear mother's father when he is no longer around to defend himself. We will not see her again.

The US ended our friendship with Kathy and Mark.

You left home and you met Niamh.

I think 2010 will be another life-changing year. Adam –
we have to decide whether to keep him at Ipswich or move
him. I think Ipswich is quite demanding. Woodbridge is
much the same. St Jo's seems to have similar results as the
states but you pay for the privilege; as much as at Ipswich, I
believe.

As an aside, Adam's friend Pankaj came for tea.
Excruciatingly polite. We even started to say 'please' and
'thank you' to each other so as not to show ourselves up.
The only awkward moment was when he asked, ever so
nicely, what the 'white lumpy stuff' was on his plate. Adam,
thinking quickly, said it was bubble and squeak. It was, of
course, just your mother's ordinary mashed potato.
Fortunately, there was none of your mother's immovable
gravy to confuse him further.

Now that Sophie is a grown-up (ahem) and leaving
Ipswich, I am hoping she will become a fully fledged adult.
The 1.30 a.m. pick-ups from Liquid, ferrying various
drunken friends about and the sleepovers to midday with
the later discovery of God knows what down the sides of
sofas, under beds and thrown out of the window for
Bernard to discover and bring back in the next morning are
just a few of the many things I hope to see the back of in
2010.

There is some talk of her and Lee going off to UEA
together; I think they see themselves holding hands and
skipping off down the Yellow Brick Road à la Wizard of Oz.

(They'd need to hold hands, of course, because they are usually both so pie-eyed that they cannot stand up straight, let alone walk.) Also, Lee seems to have failed every part of his A levels and A level retakes to date so how he is going to go from three Us to three Bs in the space of the next six months beats me. I think this one may end in tears. No doubt, somehow, some way, it will be my fault (most things are).

What do you and Niamh plan to do next? You need to be giving it some thought. I am not sure what your respective degrees in colouring-in and medieval bag-weaving are going to qualify you to do. You are welcome to stay on at the flat but we would expect to see some sort of rent from about September; we cannot afford to subsidise you indefinitely. Can you go and get what I believe are called 'jobs'? Let us know your plans – sooner rather than later, please.

Love

Dad

x

I had no idea what Michael was like, how he felt or thought, and no real sense that he was battling various forms of mental illness.

For me, things were very simple – Michael would finish his course, pitch himself and his art to as many people as he could and get some sort of freelance artistic work.

As necessary, he would, as I did, get some sort of job that he might not really want to do – for me it was part-time teaching – so that he could pay the bills as he built his artwork upwards.

Simple? Far from it. What Michael really needed more than anything this year was support and encouragement from me. What he got were sly digs and barely concealed threats and, eventually, an ultimatum. Depressed, he already faced a big black wall. I just made it bigger and wider for him to climb over.

24 January 2010

Dear Michael,

Not much to report – all is well.

Someone at your mother's work made the fatal error of telling her she was 'very funny'. (Me and Adam speculate it was someone who does not really like her and was implying she was 'funny peculiar' although your mother seems to think it means 'funny ha-ha' and not just 'funny' but 'very funny'.)

She has taken to making jokes at every opportunity. Example:

Adam: How long have you and Dad been married?

Mother: Twenty-four years. (Pause for effect.) Two life sentences back to back. (Pause for laughter.)

Adam: Stony silence, sound of wind whistling in the trees.

It has got to the stage where me and Adam have taken to saying 'boom, boom' and/or pretending to hit a cymbal at the end of each 'joke' to try to dissuade further attempts at humour. Unfortunately, your mother seems to be encouraged by this. Sometimes we misjudge a joke: your mother was telling us about Grandma's health, for example, when we did drum rolls. She felt it was inappropriate. We will persevere.

Talking old and irritating women – joke – Granny is up over the weekend of 6/7 February (it's her seventy-fifth on the 9th). We will go to the Red Lion. You two coming? Let us know when you talk to your mother so we can book the required number of seats.

Love

Dad

PS I have taken to eating soup for lunch but dare not leave the room to find a book or newspaper to read with it. Bernard has somehow acquired a taste for it, regardless of flavour. He is straight in there, licking it up. I can usually get it off him before it's all gone but it's off-putting eating the dog's leftovers, I can tell you.

Tracey was – is – a good mother. Back when Michael was little, I used to work two to three days a week as a part-time lecturer (after my work with beauty therapists, I went on to teach secretaries and plumbers a range of subjects that were incomprehensible to me and, thus, to all concerned). Tracey worked two or three days at a photographic studio and a local publisher. We took turns looking after Michael, me scribbling away at books and articles around his nappies, playtimes and sleeps.

As our family grew, Tracey still worked part-time, with me looking after the children whenever she was working. I have always worked from home, so it was easy enough to do. Tracey did not work full-time until Adam started school; even then we shared the chores of dropping off and collecting Adam from school.

Did Tracey, for all the love and warmth and closeness of regular phone calls and texts, realise what was going on? No, none of us did. By 2010, as we later discovered, Michael was slipping downwards in an increasingly vicious spiral. He had low levels of self-esteem, and valued little or nothing about himself and what he did. That, in turn, led to a sense of depression. He was almost child-like, unable to do anything for himself; Niamh pretty much had to do everything.

One Christmas, I forget which, but it was about this time, we had a Christmas card from Michael and Niamh; they made their own, both being arty. It showed Niamh as a mother holding a baby Michael in her arms – a psychiatrist would have a field day with that one, I imagine. Again, it did not register with us, other than seeming ever so slightly odd.

They wanted to disguise it from us, Niamh always bright and cheerful. But Michael, when we saw him, was distant. He had always been reserved, but now seemed to have no drive at all. He would talk normally when we spoke to him and smiled now and then but did not really initiate or participate in conversations.

Tracey and I felt increasing levels of irritation as the year progressed. With their courses ending, we'd expected a mood of activity and excitement in Michael and Niamh for the future. There was a sense that nothing was happening and never would. Tracey was better at hiding it than I was and showed a more caring face. I just became more agitated, wondering what would unfold (or not) over the summer and who would be paying for it (i.e. me).

February 2010

Michael,

Granny has been and gone. She arrived in town Saturday lunchtime. We had planned to take her as a surprise to Wyevale for lunch and a walk around the garden centre in the afternoon. But she thought me and Adam were going to the football and did not want to trouble your dear mother so she stayed in the hotel reading and did not come round until 5.30 p.m. We thought she had broken down on the M25 or A12 but I had not made a note of her mobile number so could not check. Much relief all round when she turned up.

It was a pretty rotten excuse of yours. If you knew last week you had to get work in, I am sure you could have worked around a day off. We would have paid your train fare or petrol money. We glossed things over with your grandmother and she does not give much away but I cannot help feeling she was upset by it. She is seventy-five on Tuesday. If nothing else, can you at least call her or send her a card or text her to wish her a happy birthday. It's not much to ask really.

The weekend went well enough. We went to the Red Lion for a meal; a little nicer than the usual 'pub grub' although what with venison burgers and boar steaks and what have you we mostly stuck to plain old fish and chips and the like. Lee came too and had 'the cheesy pizza' as per. He was unfailingly polite to Granny although he seemed to sit at an angle all night, leaning to his left, so I am not sure if he was all there one way or the other. There is a rumour that the drunker he is the more polite he is, and I have a suspicion that may be the case.

As for the rest of us, Adam was a bit more adventurous food-wise but then he used to eat stuff (worms, bulbs, etc.) in the garden when he was small and old habits die hard. Granny does not eat much, picking away at lettuce and what have you. Sophie is still eating for two (she's not pregnant, thank goodness, but eats as though she were carrying triplets). We dropped Granny back at the hotel at nine thirty.

Granny popped in again at about eleven this morning for a cup of tea and a visit to the toilet (as you do) before heading back. She did not want to take up any more of our day (not that we had anything planned). She doled out some cash – you have some here, as does Niamh – and was then gone. No fuss. No trouble. It all felt rather sad really. We did a cake for Nan's eightieth birthday and should have done one for Granny. Nan cried when she opened her cake. Granny would have been just fine. She is made of sterner stuff. We will do something for Granny's eightieth; hopefully, you won't be too busy for that.

It was all rather formal and matter-of-fact when I was growing up. No one really said anything about thoughts or feelings, or kissed or anything like that. Hugging was something that foreigners did. Only once did the façade crack. On my eighteenth birthday, Nan and Grandpa gave me £100 in my birthday card. I rang them to thank them and Nan, in a shaking voice, said, 'We love you.' I did not know what to say by way of reply so I just said, 'Thank you.'

I'm not sure what to add to that so I will end this here – but please do something on Granny's birthday.

Love

Dad

x

Michael had not seen my mother for some time; had he done, I suspect she would have noted the stark deterioration in his physical appearance that, in some sub-conscious way, we had chosen to downplay.

Looking back, it was probably for the best. My mother had not had a particularly easy life. Her first husband, my father, had dumped her unceremoniously, leaving her alone in a small rented flat. Her second, common-law, husband had died a long, slow death from lung cancer. Her third husband had gone the same way, the cancer spreading from bladder to brain, with all sorts of horrors in between leaving him unable even to move himself in his bed. That loss was just a few years before this. Did my mother need more heartache and grief?

My mother, like Grandpa and me, was emotionally inarticulate. I remember no words of encouragement or love, hugs and kisses from my childhood. The only emotion I ever recall from my mother was when I was about seven, just after my parents divorced. I was at my father's house – him, his girlfriend and me – when my mother came to visit me. I think this must have been before a court had ruled I was to spend weekdays with my father and weekends with my mother.

I don't recall what happened during the visit, only that at the end I walked with my mother to the bus stop and that we had to cross the road, a fairly wide but not especially busy one. We stood and waited in silence, alongside two chatty teenage girls, who, I think, must have been there to meet someone due to arrive on the bus.

As the bus came into sight, my mother started crying, saying to the girls that I was not old enough to cross back on my own and that I might get myself run over. They saw my tearful mother onto the bus – she barely turned to me – then took me back across the road. At the time, I was a damaged and indignant little boy – 'I can cross the road on my own!' Now, I see more meaning in those tears, imagining my mother watching me walk alone back to my father's house.

Another memory, from the same time, haunts me today. It reminds me of what I was like inside when I was small. At school, we had two dinner ladies who would watch over the children in the playground at breaks. One would sometimes allow the smaller girls to walk either side of her underneath her large cloak. I was desperate to do that, to have her arm around me, to be inside that cloak with everyone else. One day, I plucked up courage to ask if I could join in: 'No, you're too big.'

I was never shown physical affection in my boyhood. If, as a child, you hide your feelings behind a mask, it is hard, when you have children yourself, to shed that in-built shield and be the warm, loving parent you feel you are but find impossible to show in obvious ways.

Had my mother seen Michael in the state he was, I'm sure she would have said something to me during one of our regular, twice-weekly phone calls. But she would likely have said it in a rounda-bout way that would only have annoyed me and made me feel it was my fault. I would have been short and snappy with her. There would have been a silence before we moved on to something else, the moment lost.

28 February 2010

Dear Michael,

It's all go I can tell you. Sophie and Lee seem to have broken up again. (We have lost count too.) We never really know if it's on or off at any given time. They seem to break up. He then leaves a bottle of Coca-Cola and some Doritos and/or a bag of M&Ms by the gate with a note that seems to signify it's on again. Then they split up. We have been waiting for the gourmet cuisine to appear for a week or so now so maybe it is a permanent break. We dare not ask: it may send Sophie berserk.

Decision-time soon for Adam – we need to give a term's notice if he is to leave Ipswich. This maths business is troubling – he simply does not get the whole adding and subtracting thing at all. Remember Aunt Sally and Worzel Gummidge? They won £10 in a talent show and agreed to split it 50-50. Aunt Sally gives Worzel £3 and keeps the rest. Adam's maths is like that. Have to say it's great for me pocket-money wise (he's on two 10ps and one 5p a week at the moment). I think it will do for him by the time he gets to GCSE – maths bleeds into so many subjects one way or the other: physics, chemistry, geography.

Also, it makes him feel as though he's stupid. He isn't. I always tell him that if he takes maths out of it, he's not all that far off being below average. He gives me a look. The choice is limited, though. Both Ipswich and Woodbridge are much the same; I think that's good for someone like Sophie, who is quite driven, but not so good for Adam who prefers to amble along. Also, present company excepted, every Ipswich School boy I have ever met has been the same – smug and self-satisfied – and I am not sure I want Adam to turn out like that. The alternative is St Jo's, which is meant to be nice but a bit so-so on results, or a state school. We shall see.

I am in the wars dental-wise. My molars are shot to pieces on both sides. Two stumps, one loose crown, one filling at gum level. I look like Shane MacGowan. A dentist says he can do implants but if I have four new shiny teeth, it will be hard to stop until I have a full set and look like Engelbert Humperdinck. I am sticking with it all for the moment but every mealtime is an adventure and I never know what the ending will be.

We are going to go back to Orlando again but not the villa we had last time. I do not think it was a good idea to rent from someone we know – she seemed to ring every day or so. We will get somewhere similar for three weeks in August. We assume you and Niamh are not coming (have the dog?) and Olivia seems to have vanished and we do not want to risk taking Lee – if he is restored to favour next week – in case they break up whilst we are out there.

Doesn't time fly? We do not seem to have seen you and Niamh since Sophie's eighteenth. Should we do something before we – me, your dear mother and Adam – go away at

Easter? We could come up and have a meal maybe sometime between now and then? Talk to your mother this week.

Love

Dad

PS Just realised that Mother's Day is mid-March so maybe we should do that? Maybe see a film (nothing too sick-bag, soppy or violent, please) and then have something to eat? What do you think?

I can see that my parents' bitter divorce and the fall-out from it, two new spouses, neither of whom had or wanted children, and years of childhood misery might leave me as a damaged adult, failing to show feelings or emotions even though I felt them. I have long hidden behind humour, ranging from silly jokes to, on occasions, acid asides. As our 2007 holiday fell apart, Kathy Robertson said something along the lines of 'Iain's jokes always have a sting in the tail.' It was true enough.

I tried to express my feelings, good and bad, via humour. But as a child, I put on a face, neutral when I was small, 'not bothered' as a teenager, and kept all my thoughts and feelings bottled up inside. Who wanted to know how I was or how I felt about anything? Nobody, with the possible exception of Nan and Grandpa.

I was too repressed to say anything to them. I remember one Sunday early evening, when I was ten or eleven, at my grandparents' home in West Norwood, south London. I was about to be taken back by my mother to her flat to be collected by my father later that evening. I did not want to go either to my mother's or my father's: I wanted to stay with Nan and Grandpa, where I felt safe and warm. I wanted to ask them if I could stay, live with them from then on but could not bring myself to do it. If they had said 'No', and I think they would have had to for a number of reasons, my heart would have broken. Better to act tough, pretend I didn't care and nothing and no one could ever hurt me.

Was Michael as damaged as a child? I have spent so much time questioning my strengths and weaknesses as a parent. I also think about Michael as a little boy and what he was like as a teenager, up to when he left home and things went wrong. Surely he must have been flawed in some way or had something terrible happen to him to become trapped in the endless low self-esteem-depression-anorexia cycle that made his life a misery. Or is it that, as the terribly right-on Doctor Tom might have said, 'S-H-1-T happens'?

March 2010

Dear Michael,

It was good to see you today – some of it anyway – and your mother is pleased with the cups and bowls; they were a nice idea. 10/10.

What is it with dog films? Why are they always so sad? I have trawled my memory of dog films over the years and they all end badly for the dog.

Old Yeller – this was a Disney film, more like a horror movie, where a widow and her children way out west get a Labrador to protect their farm. Old Yeller fights off a rabid pack of dogs and gets rabies so they shoot him. Lovely. My other grandmother, Tony's nan, took me and my cousin Tony three times. I had nightmares for years.

Turner & Hooch – Tom Hanks playing a cop with a big slobbery dog as his sidekick. All I can remember is that the dog dies at the end and it's another sad one.

Marley & Me – yes, dog dies (inevitably, why can't the dog live to a ripe old age for once?). We saw this one at Woodbridge and I think we all had something in our eye at the end. Sophie staggered out weeping buckets and almost falling over which was embarrassing.

My Dog Skip – this one's too close to home, being a Jack Russell (they used the one that did *Frasier*). We've watched it four or five times on DVD but have to turn off the ending every time. Last time, your mother left the room with ten minutes to go. I followed her a few minutes later.

Hachi – why, oh, why? Who chose it? (Mother . . . Richard Gere . . . Enough said.) I could have lived through a slop-bucket romance or even a Power Rangers-type crash-bang-wallop film but this one? No. The poor dog waiting for years and years? And, what's worse, it is a true story. It actually happened. Stab me in the heart and leave me for dead. From now on, I am in charge of choosing films on these occasions.

It is a shame you could not stay for a meal. I know Niamh's mother is on her own and all that and needs as much TLC as you can give; but, when all is said and done, she may be 'just like a mother' to you but she is not your actual mother. Your mother, for all her faults (God knows, I've lived with them for years), is a good sort at heart and deserves better. I cannot help but think this is all to do with your eating thing as much as anything else. Do you eat? Can you eat? I do not want to end on a less than happy note – it was a nice afternoon, dog's death aside – but I do not see much improvement in you appearance-wise.

Love

Dad

x

When Michael was small, Tracey and I were incredibly smug parents, although we tried hard – well, reasonably hard – not to show it. Michael was perfect: he was a sweet little baby, walked and talked early, and had a smile that could charm the birds from the trees. He liked drawing and collecting things – stickers, figurines – a description that, despite everything, still fits him today.

That 'perfect' description, or something much like it, is a view of their children that many parents may have, but it was true for us. To put Michael into some sort of context, Sophie could be tricky at times and Adam was an absolute horror. He started kicking from the fourth or fifth month of pregnancy and never stopped. He always wanted to do the opposite of whatever you wanted him to do. He broke free from nursery groups, 'did not mix easily' with other children and ran off at parties and pantomimes galore. (That included his own birthday parties.) I lost count of the times I had to wrestle him out of cafés and restaurants halfway through meals as he grimaced and shrieked and threw food about for no apparent reason. It was as if he were at war, but did not know why or with whom.

But Michael was a sweet soul and, for those first few years, we could pretend to be perfect parents too. 'Yes,' we'd say, when asked (and occasionally when we were not). 'He's always like this, as good as gold' (almost purring with delight as if we had some sort of inner wisdom and instinctive expertise). He smiled and laughed easily as we threw a ball about on the green, watched Disney videos – *Robin Hood* was viewed to the stage where we could shout out the dialogue in advance – and I carried him out and about high on my shoulders, dropping him down and swooping him back up again in one long, laughing movement. Good days, for sure, days to hold on to in darker times.

March 2010

Michael,

Dramatic scenes at the Regent where we saw *Riverdance: The Farewell Tour* (they're back most years to be honest). A man in a wheelchair was cured and got up and danced. If

that wasn't enough, a woman died and came back to life.
The show was that good.

We had the usual seats, row K, at the end, right side, so I
can stretch my legs out into the aisle. But at the end of the
row in front, we had an Indian guy in a wheelchair with his
wife. I'm never keen to have someone in a wheelchair in
front of me – not because I am un-PC but because they tend
to sit a little higher given the rake so I cannot see the stage
so well. This guy was particularly irritating as he kept
bobbing about in time with the music so I had to duck and
weave to see what was happening on stage and I think it
may have had some sort of domino effect several rows back.

Anyway, all went well into the second half – lots of
fiddlers and smoke and assorted Tinkerbell-type women
twiddling about – and then they went into some sort of
routine where the whole cast is on stage dancing from side
to side. The guy in the wheelchair was rocking back and
forth by this time and then a woman, the row in front,
about eight seats to the left, slumped forward in her seat.
There was a bit of consternation around her, arm-waving
and so forth and, after a minute or two, the St John
Ambulance people rushed forward and the lights went up
and the dancers on stage sort of stopped and shuffled about
awkwardly before being called off.

So we all sat there, waiting and wondering, and some
bloke in a hat seemed to revive her and then the guy in the
wheelchair got up out of it – obviously some sort of free

ticket scam going on here, I thought to myself – and wheeled it over towards her. They got her out of the row and wheeled her off past us; she looked a bit out of it really, her head lolling to one side, tongue out, although I noticed she clung on hard to a box of Celebrations so whether it was some sort of chocolate-induced coma, I don't know. Anyway, we never saw her again.

So the show starts up and the wheelchair guy is now standing to the side, jigging about like he's in the *Top of the Pops* audience. You'd think he'd have been a bit more discreet if he came in on a freebie. The show went on to the end, and jolly good it was too, and the usher then wheeled the chair back down the aisle. At this point, for reasons best known to myself, I lurched forward to help the chap back into his wheelchair. I don't know why as he was younger and fitter than me. Anyhow, I broke the arm of his wheel-chair and gave it to his wife and then we left.

Love

Dad

x

PS All well here. Keep it to yourself for the moment but we think that Lee may have exited stage right for the very last time. Enter, stage left, drum roll, Henry Beaumont III (we think). I will write further once Sophie has told your mother in confidence and she then tells me in confidence and I will tell you in confidence. You can then tell Niamh in confidence. Let us hope that Niamh and Sophie do not talk.

Other than a brief nightclub kerfuffle between past and present beaux, this was to be the end of Lee as an extended part of the Maitland family – a shame as, over the last three years or so, he'd become something of a fixture in our lives and we had grown fond of him. Tracey and I were sad to see him go.

I often used to look at Sophie's friends, boys and girls, and, in a desperate attempt to retrieve a vestige of my youth, try to judge whether, when I was that age, I would have been friends with them. Some, yes. Others, no. But I have no doubt I would have been best friends with Lee. We would have drunk and joked and strutted about together, all of it a little bit louder than it really needed to be.

Lee went on to get A levels, a degree and a good job – we said hello to each other as and when our paths crossed. His mum died of cancer a few years later, in her forties, and Tracey wrote to him with the words of warmth that we still felt towards him. Hopefully, things will go well for him in the future.

March 2010

Dear Michael,

It's official – you may have heard already – Lee is now history and Sophie has transferred seamlessly to a new boyfriend: Henry. His full name is Henry Charles Beaumont III. (We are not sure if it is actually Henry Charles Beaumont III but the III seems fitting.) He is rather grand and Granny will instinctively curtsey if/when she meets him (thus revealing our plebeian origins to one and all).

He's at Ipswich doing A levels in the same year as Sophie. At first, he was just one of the crowd but he has been mentioned and is appearing more and more lately on his own so we had been saying to ourselves, 'Hello, something going on here.' And so it has proven. He came round on his own (with Sophie) last week and had some tea (a.k.a. 'high tea') and Sophie was at pains to say he was 'just a friend' – a giveaway if ever we heard one.

Have to say he is rather sweet and charming (albeit quite loud in a 'Yah, Father's in the Cit-ay' kind of way) and talks to us as though we are quite important; he asks me questions about what I do ('Say Aloe, Goodbye Dandruff') and what your dear mother does ('Which one of you needs to go to the toilet right now?'). He likes *Doctor Who* and Hanson (Mmm Bop) and – the clincher – knows or has met (not sure) David Tennant (at this point, I acted all grown-up and feigned uncertainty as to who David Tennant was but then realised Sophie had probably primed him that I liked *Doctor Who*). Sad though we are to see the demise of Lee, this one has some potential. The big dollop will, at least, never want for anything.

As I say, he is technically just 'a friend' but we are away for Easter – a lodge up near York so we can do York and

Harrogate stuff – and Sophie and Bernard will be taking charge of the house in our absence so I rather suspect that things may well have moved on apace III-wise on our return. More to come.

Love

Dad

x

PS You've crash-landed on the planet of the apes. Do you spend your life hiding in the forest, living off rabbits and berries OR do you go off and search for a colony of humans and risk being captured by the apes? Tough call.

Lee's replacement was a nice boy who would have fitted easily into One Direction or some other boyband. But this was a chalk and cheese relationship if ever there was one. He seemed to us to be sweetly fey and effete; she was, at that time in her teenage years, a bulldozer of barely controlled emotions.

From the start, we did not expect it to last long but it provided some moments of amusement and delight for Tracey and myself while it did. (Clearly, with Sophie, we had to keep these secret out of love or, quite possibly, fear.)

My abiding memory of those days is of dashing behind the chimney breast whenever I heard him arrive. Tracey, being more dignified, would crouch under the stairs.

18 April 2010

Dear Michael,

It is all go here and that's a fact. Sophie and Henry Beaumont III are now officially 'an item' and she does seem very happy; hopefully, being 'loved-up' will not affect her A levels. I am not sure what it is she needs to get into UEA – three Bs? – but I think whatever it is she will want to get all As anyway. (You may recall the Amberfield hoo-hah when she was expecting to get twelve As at GCSE and be carried around on her friends' shoulders – hurrah for Sophie, hurrah for Sophie – and she got a mix of As, Bs and Cs and we lived in fear for our lives for several days thereafter.)

Lee has been leaving little envelopes and bottles of Coke and cheesy Wotsits by the front and back gates – she just steps over and ignores them as if they were piles of dog dirt and I have to clear them away when they start looking a little weather-beaten. I am afraid the poor boy has his tail well and truly between his legs but to no avail. Sophie has moved on to greater glories.

HBIII is a nice boy – polite and well-mannered – but we are already starting to feel as though we are bit-part players in *Upstairs Downstairs* with me and your mother being the downstairs. He asked your mother if the condiments in a meal he was eating, as microwaved and dished up by your own dear mother courtesy of M & S, were 'home-made'. Your mother and I exchanged glances and your mother replied carefully, 'They are Heinz,' and kept moving. He asked me about plants in the garden (mostly dead or leaning ominously) as if I were his gardener. I mumbled something about having had some trouble with ragwort this winter (whatever) and he nodded wisely. I have not said anything yet to your mother but I am beginning to have my doubts about him.

We have had some drama with one of the gerbils; the light one, not the dark one. I can never remember the names or ages and have to tread carefully around these facts so as to avoid the impression that I am a thoughtless and uncaring father. Oh for the days when you had stick insects and they were all called 'Sticky' or variations thereof. Of course, when a stick insect dies, you never really know – if I recall, for the last few weeks of Sticky number twelve's life, you were actually feeding a twig?

Anyway, the gerbil ('Lighty') had a huge gash around the back of the neck, blood everywhere. We thought, originally, that there had been a fight but there was no blood on the other ('Darky') so we concluded it had been scratching itself with sharp claws. Anyway, we cleaned it up as best we could (cost of more than £10, a new gerbil was cheaper) and have put them in separate cages (which cost me another £46) as your mother felt they might fight.

I have since been dabbing away at it twice a day with some sort of salve from the pet shop – like I have nothing better to do with my life – and we are generally 'keeping an eye' on it. If need be – i.e. your mother goes on about it enough – I will take it to the vet. As a new gerbil costs £7.50 and the vet charges £22 for looking at anything, I am not keen. Uncle Franek of course – Auntie Queenie's second husband – used to take ailing pets out the back and wring their necks. But he was made of sterner stuff and my back is made of jelly (the front wobbles a lot too). I have toyed with the idea in the past of 'seeing to' your childhood hamsters in a bowl of warm water but nerve failed me even when Jamie turned see-through. All for now; more tales of love and death and misery soon.

Love

Dad

PS Sophie has taken to wearing bright red lipstick inexpertly applied. She reminds me and Adam of the Joker in *Batman*. We have not said anything – even in a seemingly cheerful mood, she can turn very quickly.

PPS Neck-wringing only really works with small creatures. Franek did it with budgies, etc. I guess the line would be drawn at a guinea pig? Imagine taking Bernard out the back to wring his neck. It's like a tree trunk. It would be a terrific struggle.

I return again to Michael, and how he was as a young child, in my search for clues to establish the exact cause of his illness, and make sense of what was going on. Sophie joined him in our family when he was four. The gap between Tracey and her younger brother was four years and she felt it was a nice one for our own children. We had vague thoughts of having four children, like our own dear queen, two, then a gap, then two more, but ended up with three.

Michael was excited by the new arrival, but when we went to see Tracey and Sophie in hospital, he was possibly more thrilled at having seen the cartoon *Fievel Goes West* with me at the Odeon in Ipswich (along with the Batman helicopter that Sophie had given him as a hello present). It was touching to watch Michael hold her tiny hand and run his finger along her cheek. Had this been Adam, of course, he would have jabbed her in the eye and run away.

As Michael started school, he made friends easily – Christopher, Alex and James – and we entered into a round of after-school and Saturday-afternoon playtimes and parties. He was never a boisterous child, climbing fences and getting into scrapes, but he was cheerful, joined in games and seemed to be everyone's friend. As he moved through two more schools, he made more friends and we got involved with the to and fro of his school life, often becoming friends with his friends' parents and socialising with them.

Michael and Sophie were close as children, still are really, with Michael being sensible and responsible and Sophie being a free and reckless spirit. They were friends with two other children of a similar age, Carl and Lauren, from two doors down and, as we lived on the edge of a housing estate, spent time with lots of local children, playing outside on bikes or in each other's houses in wet weather.

I lost count of the number of times I'd come downstairs from my study (i.e. the back bedroom) to find children I had never met lolling about in front of the television, my own nowhere to be seen. They would be looking for dead rats in the fields alongside our home or, further afield, watching cows 'doing a poo'. Simple pleasures.

3 May 2010

Dear Michael,

We braved the traffic and went to Chislehurst Caves with Granny. I don't know how many times we've been there over the years (your mother and I first visited in about 1984) but it is always good. We all had a fry-up, squashed in with loads of bikers, to start with. Then we did the tour. Then we had a light lunch with cakes. Then we staggered home full as pigs; as always, Granny rang later to say she had gone the wrong way, turning left at the M25 instead of right and somehow ending up going through the tunnel and around Bluewater before heading back out and down to Sussex. No sense of direction at all. You would not wish to join her in an expedition to the South Pole (or to the South Downs for that matter).

When we were down in the caves, the guide got his facts completely wrong about the *Doctor Who* that was filmed there (Pertwee, Mutants, rubbish). I did not correct him as it would have made me look a bit weird (especially as I was standing next to Granny, who was carrying her rolled-up umbrella (why?) and her 'I'm An Old Bag' shopping bag). I did not want anyone to think I was still living with my mother at the age of forty-nine (especially as your own dear mother, brother and sister would have eased away from me the moment I piped up).

Do you remember going to Wookey Hole a few years back (big cave, old-style amusements)? They filmed *Doctor Who* there too. The guide, who was about twelve and a half, gave a long, rambling speech about how difficult it was to film the Daleks down there – as if he were there personally – and how they had to push them along the rocky floor as they were on rollers. Quite where that came from I do not know – it was the Tom Baker story, 'Revenge of the Cybermen'. D'uh.

I wonder if all of these guides just make stuff up as they go along and it's all a load of old nonsense. 'Anne Boleyn stayed here once in 1763'; 'Charles Dickens wrote *Love's Labour's Lost* in That Very Bedroom', etc. Let's be honest, most of them could do. Unless you got a real expert turn up, no one would ever know. Must be easier in London, I reckon, where you get a lot of tourists and they do not speak much English. 'Here, Henry VIII used to punt down the Thames with Oliver Cromwell.' Anyway, I digress. We had a nice day.

Yet another birthday approaches. Do you have any ideas for us as to what we can get Niamh? It would be nice to get some perfume or some make-up or something. I am not a big fan of vouchers – we only really send them to relatives we can't be bothered about but need to show willing. And dare I venture a meal?

Love

Dad

x

PS We are going to have another go at Orlando this year (for a change) to do the Universal Harry Potter Land. I am hoping to lose some weight – something of a crash course at present – to avoid the usual embarrassment of being turned away from some rides on account of being way too fat. Either that or I have to sit in a specially adapted seat for the physically challenged where all the jolly American girls talk to me extra-LOUDLY and SLOOOOW-LY. (It makes me realise how patronised someone in a wheelchair must feel.)

PPS We have left it late this year so that HBIII can announce where he is going so that we can then announce where we are going without feeling we have to invite him too. He is a nice boy but very loud (YAH YAH) and self-confident. He is going with his father and sister to the West Indies, I think (didn't catch the name of the island). Private jet. We are doing Virgin, economy class. He said he'd never flown economy and what was it like? Your mother looked at him. Sophie avoided my gaze.

If I'd been asked, when Michael was going up to his senior school and moving into his teenage years, what it was like to be a parent, I'd have said it was wonderfully easy and it all seemed to come naturally (without wishing to sound too smug, of course). When Michael and Sophie were younger, I recall an acquaintance with an older, 'difficult' child saying to us, in a voice quivering with barely concealed resentment and wicked hopefulness, 'It gets worse, you know, as they get older. It gets much worse.' We just smiled sweetly.

Tracey and I were happy. Michael and Sophie were too. Michael was not an extrovert boy – not loud or outgoing or even a little rascal – but I could not have described him as introverted or shy. Neither could I use any other faintly negative terms such as 'obedient' or 'did as he was told'. He was just 'Michael', self-contained, pleasant, likeable, steady – a good boy. Sophie was the lively one, bouncing up and down, getting into scrapes, egging Michael on and generally being a full-on personality.

I never recall having to be 'a father' as such, telling the children off: it all seemed smooth and straightforward. Even as they grew into teenagers, with Michael shooting up in height, his voice breaking, getting acne, then bleached hair and earrings, it never seemed anything but easy. I cannot recall any real dramas, fights, screaming matches or any obvious traumas that may have scarred or damaged him. I have to search long and hard for bad or sad memories and find little but minor squabbles and passing troubles when I do.

As mentioned earlier, Adam was born when Michael and Sophie were eleven and seven respectively and was, early on, something of a character. I have many memories of his early years, perhaps more than I do of Michael's. There were certainly more unforgettable hoo-hahs. Running out of a Norwich pantomime when a group of small children in scary masks came on stage. His first teacher, Mrs Boyd, pulling him to the ground as he made a run for it as the school bell sounded. A meal in a pub in Dartmouth in Devon where, spooked by a horse's tail on display, he shouted the place down. Through it all, Michael was serene, Sophie bounced about and Tracey and I smiled rigidly, teeth gritted (so much for inner wisdom and instinctive expertise).

23 May 2010

Dear Michael,

Not a huge amount to report; it's been much of a muchness lately.

Sophie is going to UEA and wants to live in halls. All the forms are in and she just needs to tidy it all up when she gets the results (three Bs needed, should be fine).

III is on course to do not very well. When over recently, he asked your mother if she had any freshly grated asiago in stock; unfortunately not, she replied, trying to catch Sophie's eye. He did need to get Bs to get into some upmarket London place. Re-sits are expected, I think.

Anyway, she is going north and he is going south so we live in hope. On the QT, your mother rather hopes that Lee may return but I think that is unlikely to be honest. He seems to have vanished – no little offerings by the gate any more – and we dare not raise his name with Sophie for fear of reprisals. He had his faults: the drinking, the business with the underpants on holiday, the diet restricted to cheesy pizza and microwave burgers; the list is almost endless really but your mother liked him nonetheless. He was good with Adam.

We are fine about not seeing Niamh on her birthday, of course. You should have a meal with her mother, etc., rather than us. Please find enclosed a little something for Niamh so she can choose what she likes. We would have preferred to give her something 'proper' but take your point that she likes to choose her own things. It's better than giving a present she does not really want.

Love

Dad

X

PS Grandma's birthday is 14 June. Can you do a card or something, please? I expect we – me, your mother, Adam and Sophie – will go down there about then for an afternoon of hilarity unless it is Father's Day and we will do the week before or after. Either way, a card would be much appreciated; home-made is fine. Use a proper envelope and don't try drawing the stamp.

PPS This Cameron-Clegg thing will never run five years. Did you see them in the Rose Garden? It's not so much

Lennon and McCartney or even George Michael and
Andrew Ridgeley – more like the Pet Shop Boys with one of
them doing everything and the other faffing about making
shapes in the background.

There was a period when Michael's calm, steady personality might
have been changing. He moved schools to do A levels at 'arty'
Northgate School, then did a foundation degree course in art at
Suffolk College in Ipswich. I saw the superficial changes easily
enough, the relentlessly dyed hair, etc., but attributed other things,
such as more off-beat clothes, to being part and parcel of 'growing
up'.

There was an absence of girls for Michael until he reached A
levels. The first stirrings there, so far as we knew, was when we
were having a lengthy pub lunch one day and a text came through
to Tracey from him stating he'd been asked out by three different
girls that week. We exchanged smiles – 'Wonderful' – expecting
him to start seeing one, but it all went quiet again. We didn't pry.

Later, by now driving around in a little green Renault, he went
out on a date with a pretty blonde girl who was deaf. Inevitably I
made an instinctive cringeworthy comment: 'It's a shame she
hasn't lost her sense of smell as well, going out with you.' As ever,
when my more facile 'jokes' fell flat, there was a moment or two of
(possibly stunned) silence and we all moved on. Even with my
worst jokes, there was always a warm enough sense of 'Dad just
being Dad'.

Michael only dated her once. 'Are you seeing her again?' I asked, when he returned from the cinema.

'If she wants to,' he replied.

Nonchalance, so I thought at the time, or a lack of confidence? There were, as far as we were aware, no other girls until Niamh came along later.

But Michael was not completely lacking in self-confidence. I dredge my mind for bad experiences and there are barely any of note, although one still shames me. I recall going into Michael's bedroom one day feeling stressed and on edge – deadlines, a houseful of children, lots of noise – and asking him to keep the racket down as Tracey was talking to someone downstairs. I punched him in the chest, not hard, the equivalent of a clip round the ear. He said, 'You hit me,' in an incredulous tone and then, after a moment or two, he strode forward and punched me back, much harder than I had done. I walked away, winded. I'm not sure either of us believed what had happened.

We did lark about more physically at this time. I recall Tracey coming in mock-angry and laughing one evening, saying she had been over the road talking to the elderly chap who lived there. She had seen Michael and me, with the lights on in our kitchen, which overlooked the road, wrestling and falling over and getting up and falling down again. She had edged herself slowly around so she was between the old chap and us. And there was some good-natured banter from Tracey to Michael at how low he wore his trousers (I simply looked away) and one or two nipple-tweaking incidents too (Michael on me, I hasten to add). These were still good times.

Michael took four AS subjects in the first year at Northgate and we pressed him to complete all of them as A levels in the second. He grumbled a bit, mostly to Tracey, about having to do four, and seemed a little edgy, but not particularly stressed. I spoke to him sensibly (for once), explaining why I felt he should continue with the extra subject: first, it would give him more points to get into a better university, and second, he should strive to be the best he could be. As time passed, Tracey and I sensed he resented that school and the courses, and that he would have been happier staying at Ipswich School. He was doing four subjects, probably against his wishes, to please us. He got all four A levels with decent grades, and we thought, job done.

May 2010

Dear Michael,

Sensational news! Sophie has gone and got what is called 'a job' – the first Maitland child in the history of the world to do so (apart from your brief sojourn dabbing plates at the Alex). I live in hope that, one day, all three of my children will have 'jobs' and the pressure will then be off me and I can crawl into the corner of my room and die in peace.

She is working as a waitress at the Douglas Bader. I did ask her if it was anything to do with 'being legless' but she stared at me vacantly as, after all, nothing much happened in the world pre-1992. Your mother thinks there must be some sort of link to the WWII pilot but that I should not

repeat the legless comment 'outside the house' as it is politically incorrect.

She is doing some shift work – mostly weekend evenings
– at present so hopefully it will not affect her A level revi-
sion too much and will give her some money of her own in
her pocket. I think she can do some more work through the
summer – Orlando apart – before she goes off to UEA.

We have never been to the pub – despite having visited
most of them over the past twenty-five years that we've lived
hereabouts. It's one of these modern housing-estate pubs – a
bit like that one up where we used to live at Shotley Close.
Nice enough but more of a local than a place for a treat. We
have toyed with the idea of going there but your mother
would make me put some clean clothes on so as not to
embarrass Sophie and there is a fair to middling chance
Sophie might dump a bowl of chilli on my head if I did my
funny walk routine on arrival, so we will stick with the
usual round of the Alex, the Red Lion, the Indian and so on.

That is all. I hope this will inspire you and Niamh to see
if you can get some 'jobs' as well; they really are rather
remarkable things whereby you 'work' and get some
'money' so you can 'buy' things. Go Google . . .

Your Poor Father

xxx

PS I have heard the phrase 'Master's Degree' floated about
in passing in conversation this past week. I suspect this has

started from you and has come to me via your dear, simple-hearted mother. Let us not go there. It's time to get out in the real world and take it by storm, please.

Michael had continued to wash up at the restaurant until he left for Norwich, when he gave up everything – work, normality, sanity – to, we thought, concentrate on his degree. Generally, we were supportive of him giving up work both in terms of what we said and the finance we provided. We thought it was important that he got the best degree he could.

We thought we were neither cloying nor controlling parents, and we didn't want to live our lives through our children. We wanted to set them free, to fly high and low, wherever they wanted, while knowing that we were there if they needed us.

Were we controlling? Not intentionally. We wanted Michael to move to Northgate as it was arty and seemed to be the best for him. We hoped he would get four A levels for a sense of achievement and for university. We wanted him to get out there and get a job, to do something he loved and earn some money from it. We had his best interests at heart but what we thought was 'right' and what Michael thought was 'right' might not always have been the same, or even close. It's not a happy thought.

We assumed Michael would go out at the end of his course and find work of some kind. The suggestion that he might stay on and do a master's did not fill us with enthusiasm. To us, spending another two years at the same place was a waste of time and (our) money. As usual, I conveyed our thoughts and feelings through a jokey comment.

June 2010

Dear Michael,

I thought I should try to clarify exactly what your plans are as I have had some garbled messages coming back from Sophie and your mother and am not really sure what is actually happening. (I am easily confused.)

You say you cannot continue to live in the flat and that you need to move away from Norwich. Why? I thought you enjoyed the flat and being in Norwich; it is certainly a much nicer place than Ipswich, I'd have thought. Why leave? We are not saying you have to pay rent to cover the mortgage straight away but you do need to work towards that as we cannot be covering the costs of everything for everybody for ever. We could let things run until Christmas, if it helps?

If you and Niamh are going to move back to Ipswich, how are you going to do that if neither of you is working? Are you staying with Niamh's folks? You can come here short-term but it would need to be with some sort of 'moving out' target in mind. We do not want to end up with three children here, three partners, six to twelve grandchildren and what have you. We are not the Beverly Hillbillies.

The suggestion that you can't face working troubles me. What do you mean? Do you not know what you want to do? I can understand you do not want to work in McDonald's or stack shelves in Solar but everyone has to start somewhere and you need to earn some money rather than relying on me to pay for everything. Have a daytime job to pay the bills and do your artwork in the evening.

What about Niamh? I know she has talked about being a cake shop owner, lovely idea, but is there not something in between she could do in the meantime to pay your way? I imagine her degree – is she getting a 2.1? – would be useful if she were to work in a museum or something like that. Has she tried Ipswich Museum or one of the National Trust or English Heritage sites?

Has anyone anywhere actually done anything about anything at all?

What I do not want to see happening is you moving to Ipswich and expecting us to pay for an empty flat in Norwich, for another flat in Ipswich and £500 a month for the 'work' you do for my newsletters. That is all on top of what I am paying out for Adam and Sophie. I have to earn (or borrow, more accurately) all that, and the tax to pay on it, before I even start paying for ourselves. I do not want to drop down dead of a heart attack by the time I am fifty. (What's that flickering, tick – silence – tock noise I hear? It's my freaking heart creaking under the strain of doing everything for everybody.)

Stay in the flat in Norwich, rent-free, until the end of the year. Go and find jobs. Pay the bills. Then work in the evenings and weekends on becoming the next Salvador Dalí. I am sure you will succeed but you have plenty of time and you need to do something for yourselves now.

Do let us know if you are putting in an appearance next Sunday. Let us not dance around the whole meal thing any more – either come and eat properly or don't and just send a card.

Love

Dad

x

PS Norwich is not Neverland and you are not Peter Pan.

PPS I am not Captain Hook but you always seem to make me feel as though I am.

Niamh got a 2.1. Michael a 2.2. And we come to a pivotal point in our story, the moment at which it becomes clearer, via a mix of conversations and emails with family members, that all is not well with Michael.

Niamh told us, via text or email, I forget which, that Michael could not face staying in the flat, living in Norwich or getting a menial job to pay the bills.

Without him saying it himself, he had to get away, wipe the slate clean and start over. Perhaps he felt he could leave his troubles behind him if only he could begin afresh.

I was not particularly focused on his troubles: I was more bewildered and, frankly, angered by all of this. I really didn't understand what was happening and, as ever, was concerned that it would just mean more money being poured into a black hole, with Adam, Sophie, Tracey and me being pulled in after it.

Niamh, sensibly and clearly, emailed me later, setting out their plans: to move to Ipswich and get jobs. It all seemed so matter-of-fact and downright plausible that I thought it made sense – almost. I still struggled to understand why Michael had to get away from the flat and Norwich.

4 July 2010

Dear Michael,

If you cannot stand the flat any more – I do not understand why – then you can come and live with us short-term and we will either put the flat on the market or rent it to someone else. Talk to Niamh and decide when you want to come down.

We are going to Orlando, 1 to 23 August (fly out Sunday when it is quieter and cheaper and come back overnight on the Sunday/Monday, same reason). You can look after the place whilst we are away. We would like to come back to find everything is neat and tidy, garden mowed, plants watered, animals still alive. I do not think that is too much to hope for.

I suggest that, between now and the end of August, you see if one or other or both of you can find some sort of work in and around Ipswich; that, with the £500 I am happy to keep paying for the work you do for me, and a little extra (temporary) input from us, should hopefully mean you can move out by the end of September.

I think there are other things we need to talk about when you are here; you do not seem to be putting on any weight at all so far as we can see. I think you might feel better in yourself if you were a little fuller. Not eating much must make you feel light-headed. But that is another subject for another day. Let us know what you want to do and when, and we will see if we can sort something out.

Love

Dad

x

PS We want to be supportive but, at the same time, we cannot be expected to do everything for everyone. I slog myself stupid writing nonsense all the time. I would much rather be an underwear model eating grapes.

PPS Your sister has now left the Douglas Bader and is working part-time at Cineworld in Ipswich. Hurrah, free tickets! Apparently, the pay is better, she does not have to clear up sick, and when she is away, she can still work there as and when she wants, which all seems a bit unlikely but she seems happy so that is good news. Happy Sophie = Happy House.

I had no real understanding of mental illness at this time or that Michael was now experiencing it, and had done for some time. Understanding mental illness, if you have never experienced it, is, to use a trite but fairly apt expression, like trying to nail jelly to a wall. Even if you have, I think it is something that is hard to put adequately into words.

And I was, I still am, a flawed and damaged man. To me, Michael was just lazy – whereas in truth he was battling depression.

To me, he was wretched: he never did anything, never showed passion, commitment, enthusiasm or feelings for anyone. I know now that the black dog comes in different shapes, sizes and ferocity.

Had someone said to me, 'Michael is depressed', I would have laughed and said, 'Aren't we all, dear?' then told him, 'Get up and get on with it.' Easy, eh?

As for his appearance, he was skeletal, and the eating thing felt awkward and a little embarrassing for us. Of course, our awkwardness was Michael's agony.

And if someone had said to me, 'Michael is anorexic,' I'd have replied, 'Well, he'd better start eating.' Open your mouth, shove in a burger, you're cured. What was it Philip Larkin wrote about one's mum and dad in 'This Be The Verse'? It just about sums it up.

July 2010

Dear Michael,

Just to clarify, Sophie and I will clear the flat for you this coming Friday morning. We have a letting agent coming at midday. (We would sell at a loss at present so we are going to let it out until prices rise.)

We should get to the cottage by about 2/2.30 p.m. (I need to get the van back to Walton for 5.30.) Can you and Niamh be there to help us unload everything? Niamh's folks too? The more hands the better.

Please leave everything packed and ready to be picked up with the rest of the place clean and tidy. I will have to go back in there next weekend – holiday getting close – and repaint and what have you (around the window) but it would help if it looked 'nice' when the letting agent arrives.

I hope that when you get to this new place – I am happy to pay for it until Christmas, until you get on your feet – you will both be able to get some sort of work. Stack shelves if need be to pay your way. Just because you have degrees does not mean this sort of work is beneath you. I do not wish to be rude but getting a 2.2 from the Norwich School of Coloured Pencils does not mean you can laze about philosophising all day like Alain de Botton (Alan the Bottom in your case).

Work out what you need to live on – it's not difficult to add up. See what you have coming in. What's the difference? Go and get work, between you, that (at least) matches that. There are supermarkets and pubs and bars and offices to clean. Why should you just sit there and do nothing whilst we pay for it all? All I do is write and write and write to pay for everything. Your mother is a teaching assistant and she likes it but it is not well-paid. What she earns – every single penny – currently goes to support you. Is that fair? I do not think so. It's time you got yourself sorted.

Start now.

Love (although you drive me nuts)

Dad

x

The tragedy of mental illness is that it is too often, and for far too long, hard to identify and hard to admit to. A bloodied eye, a broken leg, a heart attack, these health issues, minor to major, can be seen straight away and tackled in some way. Not so mental illness where, often, the sufferer keeps everything hidden inside and puts on a brave face sometimes for years.

There is still too little understanding and sympathy for mental illness. With cancer, there is the earnest expression and the hushed voice. With mental illness, there is more likely the raised, sharp tones of 'What's the matter with you? Sort yourself out.'

With Michael, the low self-esteem and depression had been there for years, probably from 2006 onwards. It only really showed physically, as anorexia, later. And it was only now that we were truly recognising the other signs of mental illness in our son. And yet still I resorted to the same old advice: 'It's time you got yourself sorted.'

July 2010

Dear Michael,

We hope that you will be happy in your new home – it seems a nice place and village and we hope this will be a fresh start for you both and you can 'get yourself together'.

We are away for four weekends – the house will be locked and water turned off, etc. (path outside car driveway). Nikki will check in now and then to tidy post and anything left on the doorstep. There is a key in the garage, same old place, if you need to come over for any reason. You are welcome. This is still your home.

Bernard is going to a lady we found via a dog sitting service in Kesgrave. It is an older couple with dogs themselves. Bernard has been over and seems reasonably happy with the arrangement. We have told him it is a holiday for him. He looks at us nonplussed. Nikki is having the gerbils. A friend of your mother's at work – Becky Fox's husband's mother – is having the guinea pigs. There is a little boy (grandson, I think) who likes them.

I'm working like crazy at present to do this month's work and next so I can go away and not have to do anything. If Niamh/you can still deliver the work whilst I am away that would be good – it will set me up nicely for September. By the time we get back, it will near enough be time for everyone to go back to normal (although Sophie is going to the Reading Festival with Lord Beaumont III over the bank holiday – I cannot imagine him in a tent unless the butler puts it up for him).

I feel old – it will be strange to have Adam at senior school and Sophie up at UEA. She wants to go into the halls rather than the flat, which is a nuisance as we end up paying twice that way (still not let). Anyway, it's all onwards and upwards for everyone this autumn other than your mother, who is going to be stuck with the poo and wee for another year.

If you need to contact us whilst we are away – if you are on fire or hanging off a cliff edge – you can call Sophie's mobile. I am leaving the horrible thing at home. I hate this modern world and everything 24/7. Bring back quiet Sundays. I will send postcards and bring you back a colouring book. There is – usual place in garage – a little cash in an envelope with my debit card, strictly for EMERGENCY use only, please. If you do come over, water something in the garden. Make yourself useful.

Love

Your Poor Father

PS It would be good to see you both when we are back – maybe early September you can come over and we can have a nice meal like we used to do.

Michael's low self-esteem and depression meant that he had lost control of his life, or at least he had relinquished it to Niamh.

Anorexia was one way, perhaps the only way, of controlling something: his body, which was about all he had left. Everything else – what he did, when he did it, where he went – was now, it seemed, in Niamh's hands. If we asked Michael if he'd like to do something, he had to check with Niamh. To meet, to agree a place, was all to be referred to Niamh. And the time? Seven thirty, eight? Niamh again.

Of course, Michael, our sweet-faced baby, the boy with the smile that could charm the birds from the trees, could not possibly be at fault. As parents, we felt powerless. We felt someone must be responsible for what was happening, and it was easy to blame Niamh.

Niamh, we remembered, had been a 'normal'-sized girl when we had first met and was now thin. She, we reasoned, had gone on a diet and Michael had gone along with her. We saw Niamh as someone who might be controlling Michael.

Anorexia is, we learned much later, a controlling illness. It was another way that Michael could beat himself up, denying himself food to punish himself for, in his eyes, being a failure, even though he had done well with his GCSEs and A levels, had achieved a decent degree and had a girlfriend who loved him. He did not seem to see any of that. He felt he was useless, worthless and didn't deserve anything. Michael's endless cycle of self-punishment and torture continued.

5 September 2010

Dear Michael,

You may have heard of the huge dramas that have been taking place here at Hell Hole. The place has, metaphorically speaking, been burned to the ground and my body is now just a small pile of charred remains buried amongst the ashes.

It all started with the Reading Festival. You may have heard of the earlier hoo-hah at the start of the summer when I – me, of course – messed up the purchase of Sophie's tickets. I had to buy them off eBay and then go to Hertfordshire and back one afternoon to collect them in time. (Why I was sorting them I do not know.) Anyway, it gets worse (much worse).

Sophie, HBIII and friends were coming back from Reading in two cars. HBIII crashed his and he had to wait by the side of the M4 for the RAC. The rest came back in one car. Of course, when I heard this news, I asked if Henry had been 'seriously injured'. Sophie took umbrage at the way I said this (your mother said afterwards that I asked 'hopefully') and we had various door-slamming shenanigans to start things off (your mother claimed she was 'over-tired'). It gets worse (much worse).

Apparently, over the bank holiday weekend, first-year students going to UEA and who wanted to board on site had to complete and return an online form. As Sophie was away, she did not do this – my fault somehow – and so, the long and the short of it, she cannot now stay in university accommodation as it is all full. She does not want to stay in our (perfectly good and empty) flat, nor does she want to go into any of the 'grotty something-holes' that were on a list of private landlords provided by the university. Nor does she want to commute from here to there and back every day.

Naturally, this (slight but admittedly far-reaching) over-sight has nothing whatsoever to do with Sophie. Your mother, as ever on all things, is entirely blameless. (Your mother could stand there with a bloodied knife in one hand and dripping entrails in the other and it could never, ever be her fault.) The dog and Adam are exempt from blame (on the basis of an absence of sentient thought). And so, as ever, it all splatters fully over yours truly. If only I knew all the minutiae of every moment of everyone's life from birth to death, I could avoid always being at fault.

And so we stand amidst the burning embers of our wrecked lives. Sophie – will she now ever leave home? – has declared that she will have to work at Cineworld for a gap year, 'clearing up xxxx and xxxx from the xxxxxxx toilets all my xxxxxxx life'. She will have to reapply early next year and make sure that applications are 'done properly' and 'on time' (pointed looks towards me). It was at this point that I asked if that meant we'd still get free tickets on the QT for Cineworld, and the end of the world actually took place right there and then.

    Love

    Dad

    x

PS Henry Beaumont III survives. His hairstyle is intact, if not his reputation: re-sits needed.

Sophie had intended to go to the University of East Anglia in Norwich in the autumn of 2010 to study psychology. We thought she should aim higher – she'd had an offer from Durham but had turned it down. We let her know our thoughts but, as we have tried to do with all of our children, wanted her ultimately to make her own decisions. At this time, she felt UEA was right for her.

    When the dust had settled, the mix-up offered the opportunity for things to work out well. She could take a year out working and earning money at Cineworld. It gave her, with a car and money and plenty of friends, the chance to mature (a bit) before going away to university.

And, I have to say, she did mature. She became ever more sensible on those nights she babysat Adam for us. On hearing some sort of noise downstairs, she would assume a burglar had broken in to rob, steal and, most likely, murder anyone in the house for good measure. 'Here,' she'd say, thrusting her mobile into Adam's hands. 'If you hear me scream . . . or I don't come back, press 999 for the police.'

Adam, who had seen and heard this many times before, would watch her creep, quivering, out of the bedroom door, sigh and put the mobile on the side and carry on playing Fifa 10 on his PlayStation.

It also gave Sophie time to reflect on what she wanted to do and where she wanted to go. Durham, we were pleased to hear, later reissued the offer she had initially turned down.

September 2010

Michael,

I'd normally be writing to you at this time of year telling you to take care of yourself and to ask if you needed any money to tide yourself over until the term begins. This year, I think we should reverse things and you should tell me when you expect to get a job and when I can stop paying out hundreds and hundreds a month – frankly, we are talking thousands, aren't we, one way or the other? – to keep you lazing about all day.

I do not wish to dwell on things and it is, after all, 'only money' but it is my money and it is hard-earned by both myself and your mother and I cannot help but feel we are just pouring it all down a big black hole. We cannot afford to do it for ever.

I realise you are not as you should be and that mentioning these matters may upset you more but it needs to be said. But you have to work and pay your way and you need to start doing it soon. I have to say that there is not an endless supply of funds and if I do not cut it off, or at least back, soon then we will all go down the plughole. Please give it some thought.

Love

Dad

x

PS I realise that asking you out for a meal – mine, yours, Adam's – is a complete waste of time so, contrary to all of the above, I enclose a cheque for your birthday. Please do try to remember Adam's on the 11th even if it is just a card. He is your brother and a nice boy. He deserves better. But then don't we all?

These were bleak, difficult days with a lot of anger and resentment on our side. Neither Michael nor Niamh, now living at our expense in a cottage just outside Ipswich, seemed to be doing anything more than racking up bills that we had to pay. Our frustrations with them spilled over on occasions: we resented having to keep paying with no end in sight.

Tracey and I had always been pretty much in accord on most matters, certainly regarding our children. We'd often, subconsciously, reverse good-cop bad-cop stances to work out what we felt and should do. But I was quicker to instinctive anger, shooting from the hip, often without thinking of the consequences. Business-wise, I'd walked away from good deals and lucrative contracts time and again in the past because of pig-headed principles, points of honour and my personal dislike of people. I never learned (and, hopefully, I never will).

There was still contact between us and Michael but now mostly business-related emails relating to the UK and overseas property news services that I put out to investors. It was hard at times to keep things civil and superficial. Inside, I was crying out, 'When are you going to do something?'

We tried not to let our feelings show too much in front of Sophie and Adam but it would have been impossible for them not to real-ise that Michael was in a bad way. Sophie, full of emotion at the best of times, urged us at one point to cut off Michael and Niamh, no money, nothing: that would sort them out and put things right for her brother. Tough love, for sure, but we couldn't quite bring ourselves to do it in case it backfired and we lost Michael.

As for Adam, now moving up to his senior school, contact between him and Michael was relatively scarce. There was not the free and easy communication there had been. Adam's older brother was lost to him, to us all, really.

October 2010

Michael,

It's now three or four months since you finished your
courses and so far as I can see neither of you are doing
anything at all, other than playing computer games and
watching endless repeats of *Come Dine with Me*. I need to
tell you that matters cannot continue as they are. I am
currently paying out for:

The mortgage on the flat in Norwich – we are trying to
sell it (at a loss) or let it (at a loss) but have had no success
yet. (It would have been easier, quite frankly, if you had
stayed there and paid nothing.)

The cottage – quite why I am paying for that, I do not
know.

The work you do for the newsletters – this should really
mean I get two to three hours from you a day; by my reck-
oning, it's about half an hour to sort news stories and about
two hours a month to do the actual newsletters. Your
hourly rate matches the Prime Minister's.

And now, to top it all, we have what you say you need for
living expenses. I am afraid that this is the straw that
breaks the camel's back. I cannot afford it and I am not
prepared to pull Adam out of school now or Sophie out of
university later to fund you.

We will continue with these payments until the end of
December; October, November, December. Three more

payments. After that, we will not be paying the cottage rent or living expenses. We cannot afford it. You will have to ask Niamh's folks to help, get some work, claim benefits or move back here as a last resort. Let us know your plans.

Dad

x

PS Me and your mother are entitled to a life too, not having to work non-stop to fund everyone else. You can lie in bed all day and be miserable. You can stack shelves all day and be miserable. So stack shelves – at least that way me and your mother are not miserable too.

Things had got to the point where I dreaded receiving any communication at all – text, email, whatever. Turning on my mobile first thing in the morning was a time of foreboding. When there was contact, it always seemed to be the same: 'More please.' Money for a flat battery, a shortage of logs . . .

The request for even more regular money – 'money to live on' – was a trigger point for us. They eventually came over to the house for the first of what would be a monthly handout and I resentfully pressed cash into their hands, something to live on, for the rest of the month. We were driven to our ultimatum because, although we could afford it in the short-term, we saw this going on and on until we were ruined; and we would have been. They needed to stand on their own two feet, as soon as they could, for everyone's benefit.

14 November 2010

Dear Michael,

We hope you and Niamh are well. I thought I would drop you a line just to keep in touch with what's happening as you seem to have turned into the invisible man with all of us lately.

Sophie is now doing close to a full-time job at Cineworld although the shifts are all over the place. She seems to do a lot of nights to closing time and weekend mornings. We tend to go along as a family on Sunday afternoons when there is something that we all like to see. I sleep through most of them as per usual. You are welcome to come along if you like one Sunday? It would be nice.

I have had to write to Lee to ask him to let things lie. There has been some tension and bad-mouthing between Lee and Sophie and Henry as they keep seeing each other in Liquid. And, allegedly (as they say), Lee faced up to Sophie on the dance floor at Liquid (which shows he is braver or much more stupid than me as it's like poking a stick at a raging bear with toothache). Anyhow, things seem to have quietened down after I wrote. Fingers crossed.

And so we come to your dear mother. I know – better than anyone if truth be told – that your mother has very many faults. She does fuss. She is pedantic. She does go on and on about things and we do have to discuss everything half a dozen times before stopping and starting all over again a further six times. She does make us wear clean clothes and pick up after ourselves and wash up and put toilet seats down and 101 other things that we do not want to do. But she is your mother and, as my mother's mother once said to me, you only get one mother and this is your mother. Her birthday is on Thursday – we do not expect you to come down for a meal but please do recognise it in some way and do something. Your mother does not give much away feelings-wise but it is important that you do something this time round please.

As for me, more dental dramas. I had a different dentist for the usual six-monthly. I suggested she just looked but, no, in she went, scraping and pulling with the metal probe. The inevitable happened and part of an upper tooth that was holding a bridge in place came away. I could have screamed. Before I spoke, she said, 'I did not do it,' in broken English – so who else was it, then? – but I just knew that if I complained it would all turn out as some sort of race relations incident.

So I have gone back to the old dentist and have been having a range of treatments trying to cram as much as I can into one NHS band. I think I am going to have to give up the ghost on these molars and just have them out and replaced. £8,000 here. I can get them done in some Eastern European city, no doubt by some trainee student with a twitch, for less than half that. I am investigating.

I am now back to a stump and a loose-ish crown on one side and a gap and a newly replaced jawline filling on the other. I think I am going to have all four molars out and four implants put in next year. Apparently, you don't have to have shiny ones. They have a range of shades. I could have 'off white', they say; mine would be more off brown, I think.

All for now. Bernard is well and looking very furry – we will get him trimmed and tidied in the spring. Henry is still about although not as much as he seems to be doing some sort of re-sits somewhere at a crammer. We usually hear him approaching ('YAH, HALLO, PEOPLE?') and have time to hide. But he usually makes a beeline to say hello on arrival and we end up creeping out from behind the chimney breast, saying how we were removing a cobweb, chasing a spider, etc. He does not seem to think it's odd at all.

Love

Dad

x

Niamh reached out to us as the end of the year approached, saying that she wanted to get some proper paid work but feared that, if she went out, Michael would not physically get out of bed at all the whole day, day after day, and that he could not be left alone. She intimated that, when she was at home, she could create a sense of normality in so far as she could get him up and out of bed and eating at least something during the day. It made her sound like a carer. I just felt utter exasperation. For God's sake, someone do something . . .

It was also around this time that she told us she often used to read to Michael in bed – something, I suspect, that was comforting and a moment of bonding for them. With images of childlike birthday and Christmas cards in my head, I thought Michael was away with the fairies and beyond hope.

Our response to Niamh and her impossible choice – remember, we still did not really see this as mental health issues – was blunt: go get a job. Michael's life might well be going down the toilet but we saw no reason why everyone else's had to be flushed away as well.

With hindsight, and what a wonderful thing that is, we could probably have called on them, perhaps unexpectedly, to 'have things out', somehow rescue Michael and 'put things right'. We did not and I suspect that, if we had, Michael would have been even more demoralised because we had seen him off guard in such a pitiful state. It might have made things worse. It would surely have broken our hearts.

But why didn't we? I could say that it was because this crisis had limped on for so long. The drip-drip of it had somehow desensitised us to the point at which we felt constant irritation.

Also, looking at it from some distance now, there were many false dawns, moments when it seemed as though Michael was getting better and an intervention – calling in professionals maybe to take him away – was unthinkable. When he dipped, as he did often, there was always the thought that there might be an upturn soon.

5 December 2010

Dear Michael,

It's official – at last. Sophie is picking Durham (as you may already know). No doubt we will catch up on all the minutiae over Christmas so I will not add all the ins and outs and ifs, buts and maybes to that at this stage – but what's happening with you Christmas-wise? Do tell asap please.

See the enclosed photos which Granny came across and sent on this week – I had not seen them before (or at least not for so long that I had forgotten about them). I like the one of me, Granny and your dear mother all wearing the same clothes – well, dark green tops and black trousers anyway. None of us even noticed it until Grandpa told us. I think we'd all be very poor walking up and down a police identity parade as we'd been together for about four or five hours before that point.

There is a nice one of Nan holding you – you'd have been about six months, I'd guess (I've not asked your mother as she'd say you were five months and nine days and it was a Saturday at about ten past one and you weighed twelve pounds and four ounces at the time). My nan was lovely.

I remember when you were that age we would detour on the way back sometimes to see Rose (Grandad Terry's mother) in Cheam and she would make a big fuss of you whilst we drank weak PG Tips with UHT milk and ate Rich Tea biscuits (why do old people all eat Rich Tea biscuits?). She would hold you at an odd angle – your feet well above your head – whilst her brother George, who was bombed during the war, would stand there rocking back and forward on a floorboard and humming to himself. Neither your mother nor I would say anything whilst all this was going on but we were screaming inside (at least I was).

We don't have a photo of that but if we did, your mother's hair would be standing on end.

Your mother says Niamh is going on some course. Hurrah! Hurrah! Hurrah! I could not make head or tail of what it is all about – neither could your mother I suspect, but I listened to her intently as though she did – and I do not know when it starts and whether you have to pay or it is free or with a grant; do tell us more as soon as you can (unless it involves me putting my hand in my pocket in which case hold off for as long as you can). Good news, anyway. Let us hope there is more to come.

Love

Dad

xx

PS We have been to see *The Woman in Black* (cheap tickets, late birthday treat). First half was a bit of a letdown to be honest: the actors seemed to be playing it tongue in cheek.

A little better in the second half although there was a dodgy moment when the woman in black herself glided down the aisle next to me and I had to pull in my outstretched legs a bit sharpish as she'd otherwise have had to jump over them. It may have lessened the intended spooky effect. I felt a bit of heightened tension as she swanned around the back of the stage but I think it's hard to create the atmosphere when people are shuffling about and eating and there did seem to be a family who kept coughing at key dramatic moments. Someone burped at one point too. I did look at Adam but he was staring fixedly at the stage.

Niamh had decided she would do some unpaid voluntary work with a view to going on a course that might lead to a job with the council. It sounded long-winded but hopeful.

We were delighted. It meant that we would, in due course, have fewer outgoings, cottage rent and living expenses in particular, as we imagined they would be self-sufficient before too long.

With a bit of luck, we could rent out the old flat. What I paid them for their research for my UK and overseas property news services was part and parcel of everyday business expenses.

We were pleased for Sophie, too, as she had decided on Durham University, which was where we had hoped she would go in the first place. Adam seemed to be settling in at his senior school. The year looked as though it would end on a brighter note, brighter than it had for a long time.

And Michael? He was now home alone battling his demons while Niamh worked. We thought he needed to sink or swim, assuming as blithely as ever that he would, after a brief struggle, swim well enough as we moved into the new year. The idea that he might sink slowly without trace did not occur to us. He just needed to crack on, get on with it, sort himself out once and for all.

30 December 2010

Dear Michael,

Happy New Year. I hope that it will be an 'onwards and upwards' kind of year for us all.

We saw Granny today, meeting at the Chislehurst Caves car park – she'd get lost meeting anywhere else – and then going on to the O2 for the *Titanic* exhibition (just brilliant).

I enclose a couple of bits and pieces that may interest you. Maybe you could do some sketches?

It was a bit odd. Granny did not eat much and kept sitting down all the way round. She said it was backache and then pulled faces at me when Adam was not looking.

I said she would have backache after sitting in a snow-storm on the M23 for five hours before going back home. And she's seventy-five!

Anyway, she's going to the doctor's at some point; I did not press as she does not like to make a fuss. I think it's a sign she's slowing down – my nan could hardly run for a bus at that age – and we will have to start going down there rather than meeting halfway.

Can you maybe send her some sort of New Year greetings – a card or something, just to show you're still about? And do the same for Grandma too, please? (I always joke about Grandma being Hitler's ex-girlfriend but she's all right actually.)

It would be nice this year if you could maybe slot back into things with Granny and Grandma at some stage as you shape up? You seem to have been out of the loop for a while now. Maybe we can do something by the autumn. Somewhere other than the caves or Hever; we did Leeds Castle a while back and that was good, and there are other places in Kent where we can go.

Anyway, happy New Year – and don't forget Sophie's birthday either please.

Love

Dad

xx

When Michael was small we had visited my mother and Grandad Terry in Rustington in Sussex and Nan and Grandpa in nearby Littlehampton about every four to six weeks, a round trip of some three hundred miles from Suffolk. We'd travel down on the Sunday morning for the day at my mother's, then stay overnight at Nan and Grandpa's before travelling back on Monday afternoon.

As time passed, circumstances changed: Nan died and Sophie was born, then Grandpa died, followed by Grandad Terry. We started meeting Granny for days out several times a year. She would also come up to us and stay over at birthday and Christmas times.

She had tried to drive up the week before Christmas 2010 to stay the weekend but there was heavy snow and, having sat in a blizzard on the M23 near Gatwick for three hours in the morning, she reluctantly turned back. Instead, we agreed to meet up for a day out at the O2 in Greenwich a week later.

As we had lunch – she hardly touched a thing – my mother mentioned she'd had backache on Boxing Day, which she'd spent with my stepbrothers and their partners, who lived down the road from her. Tough old boot that she was, I knew, from the way she said it and that she'd said it at all, that this was serious. We kept it all nice and upbeat as we trawled the *Titanic* exhibits but later, as we drove home, I turned to Tracey and said, 'My mother's just told us she's going to die.' Tracey, having known my mother for more than thirty years, nodded. She knew it too.

2011

As 2011 dawned, life for Tracey and me was much the same as ever. I would work on my computer most days, more and more on property, and when Tracey got back from school, we would go up the town and have a coffee and chat over the day's events. We'd go out occasionally in the evenings for meals, the cinema and the theatre. A humdrum but pleasant life.

Sophie, working at Cineworld, was starting to turn her sights towards Durham. (Durham! Take cover!) We were not absolutely sure Adam was at the right school for him but were hopeful all would turn out well.

Although we were pleased that Niamh was working and now more blasé about Michael being at home on his own, there were still tensions between Tracey and me, him and Niamh, as they continued to struggle on quietly in their private hell. We were not sure what the future held for us all in the coming year but my mother's sudden ill-health was an immediate and more pressing concern.

9 January 2011

Dear Michael,

Granny rang on Friday evening – never a good sign if it's
not the usual 6 p.m. Monday call – and told me she has been
referred to the hospital by her GP. She is going to Worthing
Hospital in the next couple of days so that tells us all we
need to know (if I want to see my GP about a sniffle, I have
to wait three weeks to see a young locum who wants to call
me 'Iain'). Ray or Peter will take her as we want to play it
all low-key; if we rush down there, she will find it harder to
handle. Stiff upper lip and all that.

I told you that when Roger died of meningitis (aged
twenty), Grandpa went to work the next day. No one
said a word to him. Granny is the same. When Alf went
in for his cancer op years ago, Granny went to work
whilst he was under the knife. She never said anything
to work colleagues. Mind you, she never told anyone
her date of birth – I don't think she wanted to buy cakes
and live through the embarrassment of having them
singing 'Happy Birthday'. I can hear her in my head:
'They don't really mean it.' Anyhow, we all have to
pretend everything is normal even when they're dropping around us.

If Granny could have mouthed the word 'cancer' at me without actually saying it out loud – not easy on the telephone – she would have done so. As it was, she said she had Googled her symptoms – she has mentioned backache, loss of appetite, etc. – and 'it' (the presumed cancer) is 'late stage'.

What can you say?

If it is as expected – months – we will ask Granny to come up here with us; she can have the small lounge as a bedroom. I am not sure how we will handle things – I struggled with nappies – but we will try. I do not know when you last saw Granny? I do not want you to see her as you look now – she does not know about things with you and I do not want to burden her with it. If you can somehow turn things around in the next month or two, that would be different. It's up to you.

It seems strange that in the middle of such humdrum normality – Adam doing the usual exams at school, Sophie sorting out Durham, me booking flights for Spain – this suddenly happens out of the blue. I thought this was years away. Granny is seventy-six on 9 February and is still working, going on the bus and back to Worthing twice a week, driving up to us and back. I thought she would go on well into her nineties. Maybe she's wrong, and she will.

I have not always had an easy relationship with Granny – I will tell you about it sometime – but I would not want things to end as they are now. Things have always been rather uptight between us. It all comes from Nan and, in particular, Grandpa – they were very buttoned-up. I am told that, if they ever had an argument, Grandpa would always apologise and offer a firm handshake at the end of it. They'd been married for fifty-nine years when Nan died. He may have written a thank you note.

Anyway, not a good time right now. I always feel low at this time of year: dark mornings, dark evenings, dreary days. Not a lot of work. Tax. I'm not sure what I will do if Granny goes. Who will I phone every Monday at six o'clock? She has often irritated me and I have usually let it show. I have often been short with her. Rude sometimes (hard to believe, I know). I have not always called her as often as I should. She has always been the same though, always there.

Enough of this misery! I will write again with an update. Take care of yourself.

Love

Dad

PS If you want to talk to someone – a counsellor – we will pay for it. In the *Town Crier*, there is a woman round the corner called Jane who advertises. Maybe you could go and see her? (I have noticed that there is some other woman up the road who advertises personal services at the back of the *Evening Star*; we must be careful not to get them muddled up.)

PPS I was looking for a second-hand floor sander.

My relationship with my mother defined, in part I think, my relationship with Michael. It was not a relaxed and comfortable one. She was, at least on the surface and for all that I saw, a practical, down-to-earth woman of little emotion. I recall few happy memories from before my parents divorced and equally few afterwards as the war raged on between them.

An abiding memory comes from when I was about sixteen. My father, I think realising I preferred being at my mother's, packed up all my belongings and dumped them one Sunday evening on her doorstep. As she, her second husband Alf and I returned from a visit to my grandparents, she cried out, on seeing my possessions, 'Oh, no!'

I stayed with her for three weeks or so, an increasingly tense and strained time, as Alf pressured her to send me back to my father. He had lived with his mother well into his forties. Now in his mid-fifties, he did not want to share my mother. I suspect he had issued some sort of ultimatum as, driving me back, she said something along the lines of 'As Alf says, you'll be gone soon whereas he'll always be here.' (A spectacularly inaccurate prediction as Alf was dead from lung cancer eighteen months later while I was still knocking about thirty or so years on.)

16 January 2011

Dear Michael,

We have just got back from Worthing Hospital and can report that Granny is in good spirits if not yet up to arm wrestling. She is in a small ward with three other elderly ladies although, Granny being Granny, she is keeping much to herself.

It is, as we had thought, pancreatic cancer – late stage, a few months, most likely – but you never know. She is a tough old thing. Granny went in at the start of the week and they have not let her out again. (A garage did something similar once when I took my old Giulietta in for an MOT but that's another story for another day.)

Hospital is the best place, really. They are doing tests. I think the key to 'how long' is 'how far', whether or not the cancer has spread from the pancreas to other organs. When Grandad Terry died, it started in the bladder and they whipped that out fairly quickly but too late as it had already spread. It ended up in his brain. He finished up in bed, unable to move.

I could not quite work out what was what with Granny, but I think they are doing something tomorrow to fit a stent (whatever that is)? I think it eases the pressure of the growth in the pancreas so she can sit up and lean back more easily. Granny seemed a little confused herself and what with her mouthing certain words and me trying not to hear anything too graphic (i.e. anything below waist-line), much was lost in translation.

We stayed there for about two hours, just chatting about this and that, all very general. Adam was very good. Sophie did not come down as she was working a shift and we do not want to make a big thing of it. Me and Sophie will run down on our own – it's a weekday – to surprise Granny on her birthday. She will be out of hospital by then but not yet up at ours.

Granny is keen for Peter not to visit her whilst she is there as he effs and blinds his way through every conversation, whether it is with someone who has just pranged his car or a little old lady offering him tea and biscuits. 'Tea, yes, love, but no effing biscuits.' Granny dies of embarrassment. So that's a conversation I need to have without hurting his feelings (not my strong point).

Granny says Ray never swears. I don't think he swears in front of Granny – fair enough – but I've heard him use language that would blister paint. He's had a taxi firm and a nightclub with lesbian lap dancers so he's hardly a contender for Archbishop of Canterbury.

Anyhow, we stopped at a Little Chef on the way back – not been in one for years, since we used to go down to Granny's on Sundays when you and Sophie were small and Adam was just a twinkle. We had the all-day breakfasts as we used to do. I near enough choked on mine. It just brought everything back – Nan, Grandpa, Grandad Terry; all now gone. Adam did not notice.

We are visiting next Sunday; either hospital or at home. I will write again once we get back.

Love

Dad

x

PS It's time to sort things out. Go and visit this Jane woman – I can't remember her surname. I think it's French. Google 'Jane Counselling Felixstowe' and call her. We will pay (d'uh).

The night Alf died, when I had just turned eighteen, I moved into my mother's flat and never saw my father again.

We had known for a week or two that Alf was close to dying. My mother's employer (like my father she worked for the Midland Bank) transferred her to a local branch, and I called her every night until she answered, matter-of-factly, 'He's gone, about half an hour ago.' By the time I got there, Alan Bennett had already been and taken the body away. (This, by the by, was a former neighbour and now undertaker, rather than the writer and, you might have presumed, opportunist corpse-stealer.)

I lived with my mother for about two and a half years – warmer times. Then she moved out to live with Grandad Terry, one of Alf's friends, and Tracey moved in with me. Three years later we went to Suffolk to open the baby shop, my mother helping to part-finance it, along with various government grants and loans.

I think that, right up to the time of her illness, I resented my mother, despite all that she had done for Tracey and me. She gave Tracey a home. She helped us financially for many years. She bought lots of extra Christmas presents in the days when we were short of funds. When I was unemployed and Michael was born, our lights and heating went off in the hurricane a week or so later. My mother made a two-hundred-mile round trip to bring us a heater, food and money. The list of her good deeds, caring and thoughtful, and over very many years when Tracey and I were adults, is almost endless.

And yet I never felt she was a good mother. I remember no words of praise or encouraging comments when I was small (sound familiar?). She said once, many years later, that I was not the sort of child you hugged or made a fuss of (which instantly created a mental picture of a sort of full-sized Wayne Rooney barging my way through a group of sweet-faced toddlers). Later still, a Christmas or two before she fell ill, she came up to me and said, 'I know you don't like hugging but I'm going to.' And she did, and it was all right. Maybe it was me all along.

23 January 2011

Dear Michael,

Just back from Worthing Hospital and what a Kafkaesque experience it was. Granny, to me, seemed really ill – she looked thinner, and whereas last week she walked to the patients' lounge unaided, today she had to be helped by your mother.

Supposedly, she is so much better that she is coming out tomorrow.

They have fitted a stent – still not sure – and she is now eating and drinking again. We were there for two hours – it exhausted her – and she sipped at an orange squash but could not eat the lunch they served up. Mind you, a dried-up and curling yellow mass – macaroni cheese, maybe some sort of fungus, old socks even – is not appealing. Even Adam blanched.

I spoke to a nurse who said Granny was 'just fine' and 'ready to go home'.

Madness, really. They seem to have said it is pancreatic cancer but, from what I could gather from Granny without pressing, they have not said if it has spread or how long she has. We got the usual NHS-speak. Her 'support network' – Ray, his girlfriend, Peter and his girlfriend – are all 'in place' and so it's happening tomorrow. Lots of smiles and fake bonhomie all round.

What tells me it's all wrong is that Granny is going along with it. She is upbeat and positive – and that's not Granny. She is practical. Humdrum. Morbid. 'That's her lot, then,' is her stock response to news that anyone else has got cancer. I think she must know this is all a sham but we have to play along with it.

I should have spoken up, insisted on speaking to a doctor. Said I would go down tomorrow and take her home and maybe should have told the staff she was not up to it. Made a scene. But I didn't. It was easier not to. And I am busy. And I am a coward. I do not know if she can cope at home on her own even if Ray et al are going in daily. We will see.

Can you and Niamh do a card and post it to her when you get this? 'Get Well Soon' – you have the address? It's 26 Windmill Drive, Rustington, West Sussex BN16. Can you Google the last bit?

More next week, the start of a long saga of in and out and back and forth, I suspect. I may spend some time down there if need be. It will be like old times when I used to stay with Nan and Grandpa.

Love

Dad

For many years my feelings towards my mother were very mixed. I could not say I loved her, a shameful thing for a son to admit, but that was how I felt for a long time. Now I am not so sure. When my mother was ill and went into hospital, I was distressed and hoped she would miraculously get better. I called her twice-daily. We went down there to see her on Sundays and, behind the scenes, Tracey and I made arrangements for her to come and live with us as she ebbed away.

We grew closer while she was in hospital. As Tracey and Adam went to find food – a growing lad eats and eats and eats, no matter what – I would talk quietly with her of wills and wishes and things to do. She knew the end was coming and she spoke, as was her way, of practical matters. She stressed that she did not want anyone to see her in her coffin. For once, I did not come back with a joke.

Later I cried. I held steady as I walked into the chapel behind the pallbearers, suddenly wishing I had helped to carry her in. I reached out to touch the coffin. I held myself together as Tracey and the children cried around me. The vicar read the words I had written about her. I could not have kept my composure. I cried afterwards, as I entered her bungalow, saw her bits and pieces, trinkets and knick-knacks and the photos she had of Michael, Sophie and Adam, Tracey and myself in younger days, going right back to when I was born.

6 February 2011

Dear Michael,

We had hoped to arrange Granny's funeral this week but I've been told there has to be a coroner's report first – heartbreaking thought – and that's being sorted this week hopefully. The funeral will probably be the end of next week or the week after. The five of us can go down in the Picasso like we used to do; I assume Niamh would not want to come? She is welcome, of course. We can take two cars (your mother's Mini, I'm not rolling into Chichester Crematorium with your old banger phut-phutting and trailing its exhaust along the ground).

Shall I have a word with Peter in advance about your weight? I don't doubt he would make various 'Little and Large' jokes about us and 'stick insect' jokes about you. But it is only his way of trying to be friendly – he used to call you 'wing nuts' remember? The ears? I don't think they actually stuck out. Peter is okay.

I'm still in a daze – just so sudden. Sophie and I had talked about a surprise visit this week on Granny's birthday. Nan, of course – you won't remember – died on her eighty-first birthday. We were going down on the day – she'd been in hospital – but had not bought a present. I remember pulling into the little cottage hospital car park and going in whilst you and your dear mother waited in the car. I had a bad feeling. Nan's room – we'd been there two days before – was stripped and cleaned. I knew she was gone and just left as quickly as I could so no one could see my crumbling face. Strangely, I had called the hospital at 7.30 a.m. and the nurse had said Nan was sleeping but well. I think she woke up, realised she was eighty-one and in a bad way and just gave up.

Same with Granny. I had spoken to a nurse on the Saturday night and was told all was well. (This was despite the fact that they had had to readmit her the day before as she was in such a bad way that she was rambling about washing her knickers – Granny would no more talk to anyone about her knickers than she'd skip down Rustington high street in them.) The 3 a.m. call – a doctor's garbled message that made no sense in my half-woken state and which went to answerphone – told us all we needed to know. My call back was a hard one. We had a cup of tea and agreed she had just given up too. Maybe she did not want us to see her on the Sunday, diminished and rambling.

Anyway, I am currently going back and forth, sorting this, that and the other out. Ray and Peter are being very good. Granny had tipped me off that Ray was not happy about the will – half to them and half to me – and had wanted it three ways. But he has not mentioned it to me – had he done so I would have probably killed him on the spot. We are talking and reminiscing about Granny and Grandad Terry. Not always easy. I forget at times that the bungalow was his home too and that they lost him not so long ago. It must be painful for them whereas, for me, I have no feelings for him at all. (We were always just polite.) I smile and nod and grimace in sympathy. Maybe they are doing the same for Granny. Maybe I just think too much.

Talk to your mother about the funeral arrangements when you speak in the week.

Love

Dad

PS I don't know if there are any knick-knacks you remember from when we used to go down? Let us know if you want anything else practical-wise. The place will need to be stripped at some stage.

My mother, Maureen Gayther, then Maitland, Marven and finally Reynolds, experienced back pain in late December 2010 and was dead inside the month.

On our last visit, I had, for the first time since I was eleven, put my arms around her and kissed her goodbye. I am glad that I did. For all her faults and mine, I can say now I loved my mum.

20 February 2011

Michael,

The funeral went well – so far as any funeral can go 'well'. Other than your non-appearance, of course. If I had mentioned to Peter in advance not to make jokes about the way you look, all would have been just fine. Nothing would have been said. As it was, you made things ten times worse by not going.

What am I supposed to say? You couldn't come to your own grandmother's funeral because you had an overdue library book to return that day? You had to watch an important episode of *Coach Trip*?

As it was I said you were not well which – given it was your grandmother's funeral – meant everyone assumed you were seriously ill. Car accident? Cancer? Niamh's death? Rather than say you spend your day drawing pictures and playing computer games, I tried to imply we had had some sort of falling out so everyone then looked at me as if I had spent my life beating you and locking you in the shed at night.

You should be in some sort of institution. You clearly do not function in any way, shape or form. You do not work. What you do for me is inadequate. You seem to have no thought for anyone around you. You are very quick to send over birthday lists and Christmas lists and requests for Toys R Us vouchers – you're twenty-three – but are not so quick when it comes to other people's birthdays (Adam, Sophie) and thoughts and feelings and what have you. It's all me, me, me.

It was Granny's funeral – how dare you?

You need to get help now – see this Jane woman in Felixstowe and see what she can do. I have no idea what the matter is with you. You have never wanted for anything. You had a decent upbringing – your mother's father died suddenly when she was eleven and Grandma lost it. My parents divorced when I was eight and I spent the next ten years contending with all of that, and step-parents I despised. How was your childhood anything but tranquil by comparison?

If you do not start seeing this woman in the next two weeks, I am going to go to the doctor's and see about having you sectioned. I am your next of kin. You will get a knock on the door late at night and a psychiatrist and two policemen will be there to take you to St Clement's. You will

stay there until you are better. You will be in a straitjacket
and force-fed if need be.

Come to the house when you have arranged the first
meeting with the woman and I will give you the money for
it; and we will do it on a weekly basis thereafter. If you
haven't turned up in the next two weeks, I will go to the
doctor's and have you sectioned. We've had enough.

Dad

This outburst, which had been building for some time, amazingly
seemed to us to clear the air. Was this all it took to fix matters? We
should have said something ages ago.

Michael and Niamh moved to a high-rise flat in the centre of
Ipswich, for Michael's benefit, we were told, as there was much
more to do there than in the out-of-the-way village where they had
been living in the cottage. It was presented to us as a positive step
and we took it as such.

Niamh was working on a part-time basis which, in time, would
lead to a training course and, with luck, a proper, full-time job.
Michael took over from her the background internet research
that I used for my UK and international property news services.
Asking for the latest property news from, say, France could generate stories on just about anything from Michael at times –
flamenco dancing in Barcelona, a new plumbers' course in the
north of England, baboons rioting in the rainforest – but it was a
start.

Best of all, Michael began to see a therapist once a week. He seemed a little more smiley, still very thin but a bit better in himself, or so we thought.

We were hopeful and optimistic. Tracey and I would smile and chat to each other, taking it in turns to assure each other that it was 'early days, but things are definitely going in the right direction'. We had a sense now that all was going to be well. Who'd have thought things could be sorted so easily?

10 April 2011

Hello Michael,

I thought I would drop you a line – quite like old times – to give you something of a 'Bernard' checklist for the Easter weekend. Your mother will no doubt leave you a list of general dos and don'ts (shut the fridge door, flush the toilets, put the driveway light on overnight, etc.) but would leave Bernard to fend for himself. Hence, my notes for you.

We will leave early Good Friday and be back late-ish on Easter Monday so can you be here from about lunchtime to lunchtime? He tends to get rather tense if he is on his own for more than about four hours.

Bernard needs walking twice a day. I do seven thirty and about six in the evening. If you go much beyond that, he will sit in front of you and stare until you give in. Don't take him on. I've tried. He wins.

He has Chappie biscuits and Chappie tinned meat – under the boiler cupboards – about a handful of each. (You don't need to use your hands. Use the Thomas Tank fork for the meat. If you run out of biscuits, there is a jumbo bag in the garage, big, red, 'Chappie' on it.)

He has a treat at about ten in the evening – either a dental stick (under sink) or a beef strip (in 'Biscuits' tin under sink). If you forget, expect the staring routine. He will follow you to bed if he has to.

Don't let him on the bed. He sleeps (officially) in the spare basket in Adam's room but in his bed (unofficially). Bernard likes to sleep across the top of the bed under the duvet; no mean feat when Adam tries to sleep longways. Sometimes Adam wins, sometimes it's Bernard. I come down in the mornings to find Adam on the sofa at least twice a week.

The quickest walk is round the block – he'll do his business on the green opposite Mark Gray's house. You can go up either alleyway if you prefer, looping round and back along the high road. He'll do the Berties on the side in the alleyways. There are bins at the green and at this end of the two alleys so that is nice and easy. It's a round fifteen to twenty minutes. Don't do too much more: he has little legs. When he stops leading you, that's the sign he's tired.

Do concentrate when leaving the house – if Bernard takes charge, he will lead you to the beach. He likes to go on it, off his lead, at the ice-cream hut. You then have to walk along past the hotel to the bottom of Brook Lane where he will meet you – he has a good sniff around first and then runs full pelt to catch you up. If you let him start to lead you to the beach and you then try to change direction, there will be an unseemly pulling contest. He will win as he will lie down as a dead weight and you will then either have to drag him along as if he were a dead dog (not nice) or you will have to carry him. He is bigger and heavier than he looks.

Do not let him take a tennis ball with him. He will drop it every ten yards and sit down and look at it. You will have to pick it up and bounce it for him so he catches it. Repeat ten yards routine. This will go on for the whole walk. You will crack by the time you get to the first alleyway.

Overall, it's important that Bernard knows he is not in charge otherwise he will take control. He growls at Adam if he disturbs his sleep or tries to move him in the bed. He gives us disdainful looks at times, too, although he has never growled at us all that much. He's a good sort really underneath. We operate as a sort of coalition system with Bernard; I rather suspect we are the liberals in the arrangement.

Love

Dad

x

PS Gerbils and guinea pigs. Check food and water daily. Top up as required. If any of them peg out, remove, wrap in newspaper and leave on shelf in garage. I will sort. (Note: does not apply to Bernard.)

PPS Keep going with Jane – I am sure it takes time. The fact that you are going every week is really good and is a positive step. You cannot expect instant results. Onwards and upwards!

These were encouraging days and the tension in the relationship between us and Michael and Niamh was easing a little.

Michael was still skeletal and had something of a haunted look about him but, no matter, that would resolve itself naturally as he got better. And we were sure he was on the mend. He was engaging with us again, talking a little, showing some interest, returning to the person he had once been, we believed.

2 May 2011

Hello Michael,

Thank you for sorting Bernard and the assorted menagerie; I enclose a little something for you to treat yourself. (It's £20, receipt attached as I had a Smiths voucher at Christmas that did not seem to register in the shop.)

All well here – we are off to see the lumps at Sutton Hoo this afternoon; your mother has mentioned, with increasing emphasis and regularity, that we have not been there for a while. So we are feigning interest today and will get that out of the way for, we hope, another few years.

Your mother has worked out the cause of her allergies – it is triggered by going from hot to cold or cold to hot (an all-purpose allergy, which really suits almost any situation at any time and almost anywhere). We have been expressing amazement at her ability to identify the cause and admiration at how well she is bearing up under such an affliction. None of us laughed.

Adam and Sophie send their love. We had a meal with Henry (not coming today, okay, yah?); as always, he orders the most expensive thing on the menu – steak with plum sauce – and then tells us how it should be cooked (by his personal chef presumably). Hopefully, Sophie will see the light soon.

Not much else to report. Teeth, stomach, back are all much as ever, depressing. I think I am deteriorating by the day and will just end up as a crumpled mess of dirty clothes in the corner.

Love

Dad

x

PS You may recall the frenzy to get Take That tickets. I spent what seemed like hours one day at the end of last year flitting between TicketMaster, See Tickets, Ticket Line and so on, trying to get four tickets for your dear mother, me, Sophie and Adam to see them at Wembley. No luck, but I promised your mother that I would keep tabs on eBay – and so it came to pass that I bought four tickets (way above face value) for some nice seats towards the front at the side.

Sorted? I thought so but it turns out they are actually two seats for disabled fans – I don't know the PC term – and two free seats for their carers. So, huge dosh paid for free seats and general rip-off aside, we had to decide whether two of us were going to fake it and two of us were going to pretend to be carers, and which two, or whether we were going to kick up a stink at eBay.

Adam did suggest we all went along as Eastern European immigrants as they would dare not throw us out then. Common sense prevailed and we have taken the case to eBay complaints. Looking at the original ad there was no mention of the type of tickets these were until after the main text, about six inches under blank space and in tiny type. Clearly a chancer. I will keep you posted. We are still seeking tickets.

Better times and almost back to normal, we thought.

Tracey was happy. Sophie was enjoying her work at Cineworld and would be off to university in the autumn. Adam was doing just fine at school.

And, best of all, we had convinced ourselves that Michael and Niamh were on their way at last. There was even talk of them coming on holiday with us. Things were on the mend, life was getting better. Quite like old times!

July 2011

Michael,

I think we need to address these visits to Jane and it is easier to do so in writing rather than face to face when you turn up on Thursday. Quite frankly, I would more than likely wring your wretched neck.

If you simply turned up once a week, you could have done so indefinitely. We'd have bought it, as they say. But to say after three or four months that Jane thinks you'd benefit from two sessions a week sets bells ringing. Surely if the woman were doing her job properly, we would be moving to every other week rather than weekly, let alone twice weekly, by now.

If I held you up to the light, we could near enough see through you. You're no better – I'd expect your physical appearance to improve slowly. But you look no better at all. Your head is like a skull.

Mentally, you are not there either. The research stuff you do for me is hit and miss. Sometimes it's okay, sometimes it bears no resemblance to what I asked for. Example? Buying a property in France? Verviers is in Belgium. I'd look a fool putting that out.

If you want to see Jane, that is fine, but you will need to come over and collect a cheque from me made out to her from now on.

Love

Dad

'I don't think Michael is still seeing this counsellor.' Tracey looked dismayed. We worried back and forth, doubting ourselves, considering the possibilities, not wanting to believe. Eventually we found ourselves sitting in the car just along the street from the therapist's house at the times when Michael was due to be there. We saw her coming and going, greeting other people, seeing them out. We never saw him.

I never hated Michael, I never wished he was dead, but there were moments when I felt just about every other negative emotion you could think of. Rage and fury, disappointment, disbelief. Incredibly, perhaps, we still saw Michael as a 'bad' or 'useless' person, rather than someone who was suffering from mental illness and needed help.

But Michael was our son, and through the terrible gloom of this period, with our sense of outrage and mistrust, there still shone those tender, heartfelt memories. On the day he was born, I drove home thinking that I must be a better father than mine had been. When Michael put his first Cadbury Creme Egg in his mouth, the chocolate so large that he couldn't chew on it but couldn't bring himself to spit it out. The Saturday mornings when we'd make a packet mix of six cakes, carefully putting the icing and the Disney stickers on top. Later, the diaries we wrote on our holidays, which we have kept to this day, Michael decorating his with postcards, drawings and other bits and pieces. Years and years of good times and happiness, an overflowing pot, now dented but impossible to destroy, surely.

July 2011

Michael,

We are fine with you not coming to Spain – and we do not want the money for the tickets. (I'd have to give it to you to give it back to me anyway.) I think, given your appearance, it would be very difficult to spend the best part of two weeks on a beach. There is also a big rock-mountain at Calpe that we would want to walk up and you would struggle with that. All things considered, it's for the best.

If you have something to say to me, though, can you at least not say it yourself? I really can do without these emails from Niamh. I have put Niamh's email address down as spam with AOL so she can send me as many as she now wants. I really do not need to read these emails. I do not see myself as a bad man.

Am I responsible for all of this? I do not see how or why and I do not see why I should be made to feel bad about the way you are. You had a happy childhood so far as I can see and you did not want for anything. You were just fine until you met Niamh when you were, what, eighteen or nineteen? You are an adult.

Are you truly happy with things as they are? Do you want to come home and start over? From what I can see, things started taking a downturn for you when you went to Norwich and started living with Niamh. It just seems to get worse and worse. Isn't it time you stepped back and tried to figure out what/who it is that is really causing all these problems for you?

As you have not appeared for the past two weeks, I assume you are no longer seeing this Jane. Lord, the dead have risen and have been cured. You do need to see some-one, though. I know it causes anger when I say you need to be in an institution but where does this all end? You nomi-nally do some work for me – I suspect it's mostly Niamh, given its varying quality and quantity – and you do not seem to be looking for proper work at all.

What do you do all day? Draw pictures of spaceman rabbits? Play *Jurassic Park* computer games? Hide under the duvet singing nursery rhymes to yourself? How long can you carry on like this, with everyone doing and paying everything for you? Job, mortgage, marriage, children – Peter Pan can maybe avoid all of these but you cannot stay nine years old for ever. You need to grow up and take responsibility and just be normal day-to-day. Getting out of bed would be a start, wouldn't it? Why not give it a try some time?

Dad

PS Out here in the real world, I am still writing newsletters whilst the internet destroys all paid-for information services in sight. Your mother is still slogging her guts out with five-year-olds and their poo pants every day – all so we can pay for you to lie in bed all your life doing nothing.

For a short while, Niamh was emailing me, defending Michael. She said, not unreasonably, we should be supportive and encouraging rather than aggressive and accusatory. We should look at the positives rather than the negatives. I suspect Michael, by this time, was too far gone to really engage with us.

These were dark days and we did not really know or understand what was going on. Without telling Tracey, who would have told me it was not one of my better ideas, I decided to block Niamh's email address. I thought, wrongly, that she would assume I was receiving her emails and was reading them carefully. I, for my part, would never see them and would not be upset or angered by what I took to be criticism of me.

Of course, a message bounced back to Niamh along the lines of 'Your email has not been delivered as this address has been blocked by the recipient', which, not surprisingly, caused offence. Relations continued to be strained through the summer.

21 August 2011

Dear Michael,

Back from Spain, red-nosed and short of cash as usual,
although we had a nice time (other than the fact I thought I
kept seeing Granny everywhere which was rather poign-
ant). I thought I would drop you a line. I don't want to get
too heavy but if there is stuff you want to talk about, then
choose the one of us you feel the most comfortable with and
talk.

I am probably a poor father – I have never been able to do
the hugging stuff, I'm afraid. I think it stems from my childhood. All I knew, from as far back as I can remember, was
tension crackling in the air between my father and mother
and just keeping everything inside to myself, always the
straight face (this was before I became the fat face, of
course).

My father's girlfriend came to stay at weekends from
when I was about five or six. Hard to believe, I know. My
mother must have been a doormat. She then moved in and
we had me and my father in twin beds in one room, my
mother in a double bed in another and the girlfriend in the
box room. Can you imagine?

My parents later divorced – in effect, my father threw my
mother out onto the street – and I spent Monday to
Thursdays with my father and his girlfriend. She later
became his wife – I don't know when as they never told me

when they got married. I spent Friday to Sunday with my mother in, frankly, dire straits.

A few years later, my mother got together with a fellow from work called Alf; a bank runner (messenger boy) who wrote in capital letters – not hugely educated, not exactly Nigel Havers. He was all right to start with but hated my father so, all in all, the next few years were hell, really.

I'd turn up at my mother's after school on Friday and be told to eff off by Alf, go back to my father, who'd then take me back to my mother's and leave me on the doorstep. Not exactly a tug of love.

When I was eighteen, Alf died of cancer and I got out of my father's house. I went to live with my mother, met your own dear mother a week later and lived happily ever after (or at least as happily as your mother allows me to).

I don't want to offer this up as some sort of sob story but neither of my parents, so far as I recall, ever praised me, ever told me I had done well, ever put their arms around me, ever hugged me, ever kissed me or ever told me they loved me. I don't think they even looked at me that much. They simply did not want me.

So, I can go up to Santander to do a same-day transfer of cash when you run out of funds. I can drive to the middle of nowhere at 1 a.m. to jump-start your old banger and I can step in front of a runaway truck to save your life – but if you want mush and sloppy stuff, I just can't do it. (I would quite simply go all hot and break into a sweat.)

Who does that leave? Your dear mother will talk around and around and around and, just when you think she's done, you'll have to start again at the beginning. Adam is perfecting his 'whatever' so that's what you will get. Sophie will get angry and shout at you. So that leaves Bernard – he's a good listener and never answers back.

Love

Dad

PS Seriously, talk to someone . . . or text, email, write, send a carrier pigeon. Do something.

PPS Checking my birthday list. A *Doctor Who* picture – cartoons of all doctors maybe? – and a birthday cake, Victoria sponge, seem to be at the top of it.

Although there were calls and texts from Tracey as we went along, Michael did not share his thoughts or feelings with any of us now or at any time during his decline and fall. Shame, embarrassment, a feeling that we would not be sympathetic, maybe.

I think he wanted to hide from us and any sort of reality at this time. He could hide behind Niamh who knew all his weaknesses.

All the communication we had with him – texts, emails, phone calls – was on mundane matters as if he were fit and well. As if the spectre of death was not now pushing its way in, ready and waiting.

There was a degree of reconciliation by the end of the summer although relations remained strained, and when we next saw Michael, at my fiftieth birthday meal, he was sickly-looking, with legs like matchsticks. His skin had a deathly pallor. We still hoped that something – God knew what – would turn things around for him. We hung back, though, somehow expecting it all to resolve into a happy ending.

28 August 2011

Dear Michael,

Here we are again, close to the start of another academic year and another timely change of boyfriend for Sophie. Henry Beaumont III has been consigned to the scrapbook of history much as Lee was. Paul is now in place. We do not ask too much as that line of questioning can enrage Sophie to the point where we fear for our lives. (Think that huge explosion and inferno at the start of every *Incredible Hulk* episode.)

Having spent much of the past year running for cover whenever I heard III's voice – it ricocheted (yah, yah) in before his (yah, yah) physical arrival in the (yah, yah) house – I had something of a pleasant conversation with him recently. He wanted to know the best place for his father to buy a house for him in London for his university studies (?! suffices for one of those face things, mouth open). We also had a somewhat surreal conversation about Hanson, who are at the O2 (small bit) later in the year. To my horror, I came close to asking him if he'd like to come with me to see them but then had a terrible mental image of this bloated old man shuffling in with this beautiful but slightly effete Adonis and how it might look to others. Anyway, next thing we know he has gone just as quickly as he arrived.

We do not know much about the new one yet but I expect he will be more Shaggy than Fred. I got a call from Sophie one afternoon when she was out with Lulu and, she said, two lads and she then started asking me odd questions about myself, which aroused my suspicions immediately. (I think she was trying to get me to say 'fairly flexible', probably to win some sort of bet.) Anyway, that, combined with a slight echo, made me realise I was on some sort of loudspeaker so everyone could hear me. I asked which of 'the lads' was hers and what his father did for a living and she said I was weird and rang off. Job done. We await his arrival – we have some score cards (0 to 6) from the last *Dancing On Ice* tour programme – we may utilise those at our meeting if he looks a good sort.

We will invite him to my fiftieth birthday meal – we think we should go somewhere different and a bit nicer than the Alex or the Red Lion as it's the beginning-of-the-end birthday so your mother has suggested the Butt & Oyster, which is meant to be nice but a bit fishy. Can we have a nice meal together? It would be good to have everyone there. We may possibly tell this Paul about our UFO experience so it is well worth coming for that.

Love

Dad

x

PS I had not realised, until I saw the holiday photos, that I now have a bald patch to add to all my other woes. With the first two or three pictures – me in the sea at Calpe with my back to camera – I thought it was some sort of camera effect, a bit like red eye. I then mentioned it in passing, very casually, and your mother and Adam both said in unison, having obviously colluded for this moment in time, 'We know, we did not like to mention it.' I don't know where I go from here – billiard-ball bald, I imagine. It is all too much at times.

As with Lee before him, we grew to like Henry, despite my silly jokes, but it was always an 'odd couple' type of relationship that was never going to last. He was unfailingly polite and friendly, went out of his way to chat and show interest in us and what we were doing, and I don't doubt most parents would have been delighted to have him as a future son-in-law. He was certainly a good-hearted soul but his languid charms were not right for Sophie – our big, bouncing psycho Tigger – so we were not unhappy to see him go.

There was a lot of discussion between Tracey and myself as to what the new boyfriend might be like – dashing, charming, with some get-up-and-go – and whether he might be 'the one'. He joined us for a birthday meal where all seemed well, a nice enough lad who listened carefully as I told him about the UFO that had hovered alongside our block of flats years ago and explained that we had not been taken up in the craft on that occasion. Everyone else had heard the story many times before, of course. He seemed slightly bemused. Tracey struggled not to laugh and failed badly.

18 September 2011

Dear Michael,

A brief line just to update you on 'love and romance' developments here at Chez-Madhouse.

Bring back HBIII, all is forgiven. Sophie is already besotted with the latest boyfriend, 'the halfwit', and is very sensitive about him as I unfortunately referred to him as such in conversation with your mother when Sophie was earwigging from the stairs.

We are trying to be positive about him. The fact that he works in a sweet shop and still lives at home with an aunt (well into his twenties) is not a promising start. He had been presented to us, pre-meeting, as some sort of derring-do adventurer. He is more Mr Bean.

What's worse is that he is by some way the most boring man we have ever met in our lives. He has absolutely no topics of conversation and spends most of his time staring into space. Your mother thought at first he might be doing some Einstein-style, Big Bang, Theory of Creation-type calculation in his head. But he seems to be in a permanent daze as if he has wandered away from some terrible car wreck on the M25.

All of that is, apparently, beside the point. He is nice to Sophie and, I am told, that is all that matters. (Why not get a gerbil for company instead?) Whether she will say that in twenty years' time, when he will still work in a sweet shop and they will live in a one-bed mid-terrace with three snot-nosed kids and a Y-reg 103 is another matter. Perhaps I will be dead by then and this can become Halfwit Towers.

Anyway, she is off to university soon so hopefully that will bring matters to a swift end. We have seen, with both Lee and HBIII, that Sophie has a killer instinct when it comes to ending relationships so we live in hope. There is some talk of another meal – maybe a Chinese at home – before she goes. I think Sophie will want the halfwit to be there too. Sit next to him and try to find something to talk to him about. God knows it's not easy. I've tried.

Love

Dad

x

PS Some houses have really inappropriate names. I drove into Colchester the other day – long story, your mother, Laura Ashley – and there was a big ugly block of flats on the way in. Its name? Brick Hell? Monstrous Dump? Crap Hall? No – Orchard View, yet all you could see from it were roads and traffic.

My relationship with Sophie is another story for another time but, as with our two boys, we adopted a laid-back approach. Billy Crystal's comment, 'My daughter can have sex, but only when I'm dead', is, in my view, a terrible thing to say (Sophie would be fifty-seven). Another American comedian – it may well have been Billy Crystal again – has said that he would greet each prospective beau with the words, 'Treat my daughter well. I've a shovel out back. The hole is dug. Ain't no one going to miss you.' That, too, strikes me as rather unreasonable. All I would say is that there isn't a man out there who is good enough for my daughter, which seems perfectly fair and reasonable to me and, I suspect, most fathers.

I mention this because, having been through two boyfriends, we were now presented with a third and my tongue-in-cheek comments about him – he wasn't really half-witted or incredibly boring – should be seen in this context.

Even so, we knew early on, no *Dancing On Ice* scorecards needed, that Paul and Sophie were another mismatch, even though, despite my inane comments, we could see he was a genuinely nice person and meant no harm. My jokes really boiled down to the fact that, like Henry before him, this one would not last that long.

Paul, quite simply, was someone who seemed to us to amble along, happy with his lot. (Nothing wrong with that.) Sophie was driven and wanted to be the best she could be. These two extremes do not often sit together easily.

Sophie is the girl who had spent a lunchtime crying in Christchurch Park in Ipswich because she got three A grade A levels. These were not tears of joy but of frustration that she had not got the three A*s she had been hoping for. (A rare word of advice: always think twice before congratulating a high-flier on three As when higher grades are available.)

25 September 2011

Dear Michael,

Halfwit news report.

You seemed to do well with the halfwit. I did not get a chance to ask you what you talked about. I have tried football (he doesn't like sport) and cars (he does not drive) and cooking (he survives on take-outs, I believe).

Your mother, who is woefully out of touch, attempted a dismal conversation about the latest hit parade, all to no avail. He answers every question you put to him perfectly politely but does not then take the conversation further. It ends up like something off *Mastermind* where most of his answers amount to 'pass'. Adam says he likes games where you kill people. I did not want to discuss that over dinner.

It gets worse. He stayed over the other night. He reminds me of Bernard, who lies down in the long grass and thinks you cannot see him if he cannot see you. The halfwit comes in at about eleven when we're on the nod and creeps his way upstairs without a word. He then waits until I have set off to take Adam to school the next morning and slips out.

Of course, the other night, Adam was off sick (nothing much: he had just taxed his brain too much and it over-loaded). As the halfwit slipped through the kitchen on the way out, he found me sitting there smiling sweetly at him. One-nil to the old fellow, I think. He tells me he is thinking of training to be a solicitor. I think he's too dull and boring.

End of news report.

Love

Dad

xx

PS The BBC reports that two children adopted by separate families as babies married and have just found out they are actually brother and sister. I rather suspect they might be the halfwit's parents but I have not asked Sophie. I do not wish to pry unduly.

Sophie was off to Durham shortly and, with new friends, new experiences and new watering holes awaiting her, we felt sure this would spell the death knell for her and Paul as a couple.

Surely, with him in Ipswich and her in Durham for much of the year, a four- or five-hour car journey or train trip via Peterborough and various northern hotspots, they would not stay together in some sort of long-distance relationship. Would they? Dear God, it couldn't last for ever, could it? He wasn't 'the one', was he?

October 2011

Dear Michael,

Hello, I thought I'd drop you a line what with your birthday approaching – see enclosed.

We've just returned from offloading Sophie at Durham; the four of us left yesterday morning and stopped at Sherwood Forest mid-morning and arrived at lunchtime. Obviously, as 'the world's most embarrassing parents', we had to clear off pretty much straight away and spent most of the weekend in downtown Darlington. Returning to check all was well this morning, we found a note saying she'd gone off with (all her new) friends to the pub, so we slunk back home, arriving mid-afternoon. I feel like a taxi driver who was expecting a big tip and ended up wiping vomit off the back seat.

Weekend highlights? There was some trepidation as to what her room-mate Olivia would be like – the posh-London/Suffolk-yokel contrast was feared – but they seemed to hit it off at first sight. She is quite smiley and bouncy and is doing theology. She said she had a big Bible that should prove useful for propping the door open in hot weather. So she has a good sense of humour anyway. It will stand her in good stead in the year ahead.

I thought I should break the habit of a lifetime and actually kiss Sophie goodbye as there were some people milling around. She recoiled as if I had brandished a knife. So I won't be trying that again any time soon. Your mother managed to kiss her after a brief tussle – your mother is quite determined in these affairs. Adam looked in the opposite direction throughout as if he were somewhere else.

The hotel was fine. We all squeezed into one room, with Adam on some sort of camp bed. I had to tell him off for larking about with the tea and biscuits at one point and then sat down on his camp bed, which promptly gave way with my backside wedged between two slats. Cue howls of laughter from Adam and your mother. Eventually, they helped extricate me from the bed and we managed to patch it up. For future reference, never sit on the middle of a camp bed, taking it by surprise. Instead, approach it side on and add weight evenly and carefully.

We ate at some Darlington pub-type place in the evening. It did not have cutlery chained to the table but it had that sort of ambience. I think the Krays would have run scared. Various shaven-headed and tattooed people sat around, elbows on table, swilling down bottles of lager and the like (that was just the women; not a Babycham in sight). We sat there in near silence hoping no one would pick a fight with us.

The steaks were about a fiver each so I dread to think which animal they came off, let alone which part. We were asked to leave at 9 p.m., not because of any unruliness or loudness on our part but because Adam is under sixteen. We missed our £2.99 puddings, which may just have been the highlight of our day. The tattooed woman next to us downed two without deviation, possibly some sort of '2 for 1' offer.

Anyway, we are back home safe and sound now – I can't say it was quite the weekend we had expected but we don't do much in the way of emotion, as you know, so all things considered, it was okay. There is some talk of Sophie coming down or us going up sometime between now and Christmas.

How are things? I enclose a cheque for your birthday – it's in the card (if you haven't opened it already) so you can buy what you want. If you fancy a meal for your birthday do let us know. We are happy to do something somewhere, sometime. It would be good to keep things going along.

Love

Dad

PS Please remember Adam's birthday on the 11th. He likes the BBC *Merlin* show; there's a magazine just out. Maybe a figure for his windowsill? If you have no money, draw him a picture. There will be a Pizza Hut meal – B&Q not Copdock.

We had experienced some torrid times in 2011: my mother's death, the issue of the visits to the therapist, and Michael and Niamh deciding they would not come on holiday with us. These had stretched relations to breaking point. We did not want to risk severing them completely so, despite the problems, we tried to keep things nice and jolly-ish and left them to their own devices.

Still seeking that elusive peace of mind and happiness, Michael and Niamh had moved from Norwich to Ipswich in the summer of 2010. Then, in 2011, they moved twice more, first to a high-rise block of flats in Ipswich, a tiny, cramped, soulless place where drug-dealing and prostitution were rife, and then to a maisonette on a road close to the railway station where they seemed to settle for a while.

They put a brave face on for us with their various comings and goings but these were desperate days for Michael, with Niamh trying to build some sort of income for them both. Depressed, at home on his own, with no work for more than a year and very little money, he sank to his lowest point.

20 November 2011

Dear Michael,

Thank you for coming to your dear mother's meal – I am not sure what was most moving: you and Niamh coming, Sophie turning up out of the blue from Durham, the half-wit appearing out of the shadows or the cost of paying for the meal. Anyhow, it is getting to be quite like old times.

I was wondering if you'd like to do some more work for me if you are short of cash and have some time on your hands? The newsletters are still ticking along, although I think their days are numbered what with the internet and all, so I have been developing the property news information service somewhat. I need someone to gather up assorted news and views on America and Spain, etc., for weekly round-ups. It will free up my time to do more UK stuff and to source deals to introduce to members and pay the bills. Let me know?

It was good to hear that Niamh is now on this course; I did not really quite understand what it is all about other than it is some sort of on-the-job training. Bit of a journey. I assume if all goes well that the council might offer her a proper job at the end of it? That would be wonderful.

How are you doing money-wise at the moment? I do not imagine the £500 we pay you goes too far? Do you get any

benefits or are Niamh's folks helping out? Keep us in the
picture. We could assist a little bit if need be.

   Love

   Dad

PS Small steps are all you need to take. One step at a time.
One day, you will suddenly realise you've come some
distance.

We could not bring ourselves to push Michael hard about him and
Niamh, whom we still saw as being a possible cause of his down-
fall. If we confronted Michael, forced him into a 'her or us'
scenario, we would lose him to her for ever. We had no doubt
about that. This was a fear that we had had for a long time and I
think it was as much a reason as anything else for us holding back
when we possibly should have moved in.

   Both Tracey and I had 'form' as they say. My own childhood
memory of my mother choosing Alf over me when I was sixteen,
the long drive back to my father's, sitting in silent rejection, was
haunting. Tracey had, at the age of seventeen, following troubled
times with her mother, left home to live with me. They did not see
each other for more than twenty years, until a chance meeting
between us and a long-forgotten family member triggered an unexpected reunion.

   We could not bear to risk losing Michael, leaving him to his
fate. At best, perhaps we'd not see him for twenty years. Not see

him marry, go to work, have children and, eventually, a contented life. Tracey's mother hadn't known of Michael, Sophie and Adam's existence until they were fifteen, eleven and four. It was unthinkable that that could happen to us. We couldn't face it. So we grumbled and groaned between ourselves but kept as quiet with them as we could.

December 2011

Dear Michael,

I thought it would be nice to bring you up to speed with family matters before Christmas. Will we see you at some point over Christmas time? We have panto tickets for both of you Christmas Eve morning.

We are going to move Adam from Ipswich to Woodbridge or St Joseph's. Ipswich have been nudging us gently but firmly towards the exit door for the past few months with various emails and reports to suggest Adam is off the pace by some distance. The school caretaker's dog beat him – albeit only just – in the recent maths test. It's all As and Oxbridge applications there these days. You can't stare out of the window with your finger up your nose any more.

We have been called in for a meeting with the head of the lower school and the new headmaster 'who wishes to be present'. On the basis that it's better to jump than be pushed, however sweetly it is done, we have arranged visits to Woodbridge and St Joseph's. We don't need to sit there listening to the latest educational gobbledygook to tell us that Adam needs to leave. I suspect it will be St Jo's – Woodbridge seems similar to Ipswich in the endless drive for grade As all-round.

Granny's bungalow has now been sold and I have been clearing it out at long last with Ray and Peter. It was a soul-destroying experience, having to pick through Granny's half-used bottles and potions in her bathroom cabinet. There was a small coffee-table in the garage that she and my father must have been given for their wedding back in 1957/8. I remember, when I was about five or six, crawling below it pretending I was Jamie in *Doctor Who* escaping from the Daleks through a cave. Peter dragged it out into the drizzling rain and broke it up with some sort of kung-fu kick, then jumped up and down on it before throwing it into the back of his van. A life broken up, bin-bagged and dumped all within three and a half hours. Peter then took us for an effing Big Mac.

I've lost count of the number of times I've been down there this year for this, that and the other. When I drove back this time, I remember leaving and I remember getting back home but I don't remember anything in between. I usually take a stack of CDs with me – REM, etc. – and play them loud both ways (your mother disapproves and does that sniffing thing). This time, I did not listen to one. I do not remember the Dartford Tunnel at all nothing. Automatic pilot all the way. Never experienced that before.

Your mother is gearing up for Christmas by writing 100s of cards. The hallway will resemble Clintons come Christmas. I usually get about three cards as you know – a completely blank one from a business called MBI (no idea who they are but they send an unsigned one every year), another from a guy called Bill from Portsmouth (we met on a *Fugitive* online forum* and he later met and married a woman called Julie who turned out to be about ten years older than she first claimed and he was very angry about it) and one from a fellow called Nick Daws, who wrote articles for me at Fleet Street about ten years ago. Sad, really.

Your mother has to do something with this year's Christmas production at the school. Last year's was memorable. The parents were meant to get there at six thirty but all turned up at six so teachers and other staff had to fight their way through the mob. It turned ugly. Several children were sick, inevitably. *Swallows and Amazons* days.

Sophie is back for Christmas next weekend as you may know. We are 'lying low' and not mentioning Christmas to her as, out of politeness, we feel we would need to invite the halfwit but do not really want to. Based on previous form, he'd sit there staring vacantly as we open the presents, vacantly as we have dinner, vacantly as we play games in the afternoon. You might as well put a log against the wall.

At least it would give Bernard something to cock his leg against.

It would be good to see you at Christmas – Eve, Day or Boxing. Surprise us and turn up at the Wolsey at 10 a.m. on Christmas Eve! We can take things from there. Your mother will cook loads. You can help us eat it. Or just watch . . .

Love

Dad

PS *It talks about the 1960s TV series. Bill is not some sort of man on the run. He cleans the toilets on Portsmouth seafront and was mugged a year ago as he was leaving. The mugger ran off with his toilet accessories (bleach etc.).**

PPS ** I know this sounds a bit like that old joke about the police having their toilet stolen and having nothing to go on but it is all true.

PPPS We are off to Grandma's next Sunday – sadly, no more tricky arranging of Granny one weekend and Grandma the next any more – and will report back. She will no doubt have got you and Niamh something so can you reciprocate in some way, shape or form? If you could send a card before next weekend, we can comment on it when we arrive and say how busy you are all the time (as if). No doubt Grandma will buy me the usual 'intelligent' book, which I will be unable to understand at all.

We tried hard to keep things from Sophie and Adam as much as possible, especially Adam. We knew Sophie was a robust human being but Adam, only nine when Michael went away, was growing up and you never really know what's going on inside a child at that age or how he or she will turn out. We had little or no family to turn to. No kindly uncle. No interested aunts. Our best friends had long gone. Spending thirty years writing in your bedroom is not conducive to close friendships. Tracey talked to friends at work, always ending up back in the same place, unsure what to do. And we talked to each other, of course, horrified that our laissez-faire style of parenting had led to this sorry state of affairs.

I did, at some stage in this blur of a year, pluck up the courage to go to our GP's practice. I went with some reluctance as I was not really expecting much assistance from the new young doctor I sat in front of early one morning.

Me: 'Um, it's my son. I'm really worried about him.'

GP: 'Okay, what's his name?'

Me: 'It's, er, Michael, Michael Maitland. I'm not sure what to do.'

GP (presses various buttons on her computer): 'He's not registered at this practice.'

Me: 'I need to do something.'

GP shrugs (in indifference, or so it seemed to me at the time, in my highly charged state).

I walk out.

I did not want to have Michael sectioned, a horrifying thought, but I needed someone to talk to who might be able to help us in some way. A shoulder to lean on, if not to cry. Put off, we left the practice and did not approach the NHS again.

We discovered later that Michael and Niamh too had spent much of this year and the last one, moving from one GP to another to try to find someone who understood what was happening with Michael and could offer assistance. Much of it came in the form of tablets, which Michael did not really want. That search for a more holistic and lasting solution was to continue long into 2012 without success. Like us, those wretched GPs failed him as he sank further into the abyss.

2012

At times over the years, there had been seven of us sleeping regularly under the one roof, more on occasions with sleepovers and such. It had always been a lively and vibrant house. Now, there was just Tracey, Adam and me, plus Bernard (and various gerbils and guinea pigs coming and going on a never-ending wheel of death). We appreciated the peace and quiet as we all got along well together without drama or mishap.

We kept in close touch with Sophie up at Durham, with daily texts and chats between her and Tracey. I spent many Monday mornings queuing at the post office to send Sophie a Jiffy-bag full of bits and pieces; make-up, hand warmers, chocolate treats, the odd winning scratch card. She would reappear often, popping up at birthdays, when her old school closed down unexpectedly, and for holidays, of course. Paul would rarely be more than a few minutes behind her.

Niamh was still out working, trying to kick-start a new life for them, Michael stuck in his prison of self-contempt and loathing, not eating to punish himself and make himself feel even worse. Not really knowing what to do and with NHS help seeming useless, we came to the unspoken conclusion that 'what will be will be'. Even at this late stage, we thought Michael would turn things around on his own and come good.

January 2012

Michael,

Groan – here we are again, another dreary start to another year. We – me, your dear mother, Sophie and Adam and Bernard – have all set New Year resolutions.

Me – One way or the other, I've been doing these how-to newsletters and reports since 1997 and that's a good run, given the impact of the internet on information publishing. It's killed it, really. It's hard to see it lasting much longer and I cannot go back to writing how-to books as those only sell at twopence ha'penny a time to obscure African states. We must do more with the free property news services and introductions off the back of them; we will do some extra weekly emails on different markets, etc. Are you up for some more work (and a little bit more money)? I think we need to tackle Facebook and Twitter and maybe blogs, etc., God help us. Where do we start with all of that? Can you do some apps?

Your mother – We have just started the annual diet as your mother has decided we are both too fat. I have tried the 'You're not fat, you're short' routine to little effect. Your mother says she cannot fit into her clothes and it troubles her. I say I can't either, but it's never bothered me. We will persevere for a while until your mother's trousers fit again. I have been swimming thirty to forty-five minutes every day Monday to Friday and eating a sensible breakfast, lunch and dinner for ages now but still stay the same (jumbo) weight. Your mother thinks it may be my glands. I think it's what I eat in between meals but do not say too much about that side of things.

Sophie – Apparently, Sophie has to get a 2.1 from Durham University OR ELSE it's all a COMPLETE WASTE of time (cue more dents from head-butting the kitchen boiler if she gets a 2.2). I do not really understand what's what in academic circles (me with my CSE in sociology) but this year is a 'free year', and as long as she passes she continues to the second year and this year does not count towards the final mark. Next year does – 40 per cent of the total, and she needs to get 60 per cent overall to get a 2.1. I think. All a bit bewildering. Perhaps you can explain it to me some time.

Boy Wonder – Incredibly, Adam is starting St Jo's in all the top sets from what I can make out. He was in pretty much all the bottom sets (for maths, he was near enough down and out on his own). I vaguely recall reading about Albert Einstein doing badly at school because they did not recognise his level of genius. Is history to be repeated? Is the name 'Adam Maitland' destined to be known worldwide, fêted by kings and presidents, honoured by the Nobel Prize, or is it all a big mistake and he'll end up spending his days shuffling empty boxes back and forth in a storeroom to kill time? I wonder . . .

Bernard weighed in at the vet at about 10.5 kilograms on the latest check-up, which is about 0.5 over what he should be for his size. 'He's a big lad,' said the vet. 'Aren't we all?' I replied, trying to be light and amusing. She looked a bit put out. I thought it best not to dig a deeper hole so I just kept quiet.

So, slightly longer walks morning and evening, just one snack a day (night-time) and a few more garden larks to keep him active. He cannot lie about all day in the orangery and keep eating willy-nilly. (Every time I go in the kitchen he follows me through hoping for a snack.) How he will take to all this, I dread to think – there may be trouble ahead. We will have to sneak it up on him slowly so he does not notice.

What are your plans for 2012? Hopefully, you can sort yourself out and get a job soon. What about these Game-type places in town – a good way to play games all day and get some money? We will continue with the money each month for the work you do for me until you are self-sufficient; hopefully 2012 not 2042. I do not want to be writing this 'How to Free Your Lifeforce with a Head Massage' nonsense into my grave.

Keep us posted.

Love

Dad

PS We are going to Orlando again in August, the first three weeks. We do not imagine you will want to come as we know Niamh struggles with the long flight and heat. You are welcome, though, if you want, but you will need to let us know now whilst I can get flights at reasonable prices. The halfwit is to join us.

After fifteen years, 2012 marked the end of my days writing hard-copy newsletters for a range of publishers across the UK.

I had worked originally for a publisher called Fleet Street Publications back in 1997 and edited a newsletter, *Personal & Finance Confidential*, with a healthy monthly circulation of about 20,000. Through Maple Marketing and Streetwise Publications, with the usual fall-outs and bust-ups along the way, I finally edited a newsletter called the *Streetwise Bulletin*; I suspect this ended up with a circulation in the low four figures, if that. From where I was sitting, the internet had killed off most of such publications.

I was not unduly concerned at its demise even after so many years: no mid-life crisis for me. I didn't really have the time or the energy for that. Anyway, my online property news services had by now replaced and surpassed hard-copy newsletters as a source of income. In many ways, my life – back bedroom, desk, computer, staring vacantly into space, talking to the dog – continued as it had ever done.

April 2012

Michael,

I thought I would drop you a line to clarify our thoughts about your living arrangements. Ideally, if you and Niamh can find a place between now and when you have to move out that would be best all round. Go forward, never back. If you need a financial top-up between that point and Niamh earning money from September, we can assist but please do not ask unless you really need it. We still have Adam's fees (more than Ipswich), plus Sophie's Durham flat, etc., and your earnings too; it all adds up. There is no money tree at the bottom of the garden.

Bottom line, you can both move in here on a short-term basis until the autumn, if need be. You would need to go in Adam's old room as we do not want to have to move him out of your room. We will help as best we can but Adam stays put.

If you move back, you would need to be normal (or at least try your best). You'd need to get up at the same sort of time as the rest of us – 6.45 to 7.15 a.m. – and not lie in bed all day staring at the ceiling. Me and Bernard have a daily routine – I work, he lies in the sunlight in the orangery, we meet at lunch when he stares pointedly at my food, shaking. I don't want that disrupted too much. I'd expect you to get out and about instead of just sitting there all day. Obviously, you and Niamh can sort out your own wacky-backy food in the evenings but it would be nice if we could sit down and share our day's experiences at least sometimes anyway. We'd like to see you eat. Can you manage that?

In some ways, it might be good if you were here when we went to Florida – it might stop burglars breaking in and trashing the place. Then again, we may come back and find the burglars would have left it nicer than you do. Obviously, I accept that when we get back the plants will all be dead, the grass will be three feet high and the rubbish will be piled up. But can we keep the indoors straight and the dog alive that long? And the gerbils and the g-pigs? That would be good.

Have a talk with Niamh and let us know? We can prob-ably sort a van for you – the halfwit's uncle has a van. We can probably get your stuff into the garage if we move things around a bit. Me and Sophie can do it, as we did for Norwich; I assume neither you nor Niamh can lift anything. (We are not carrying you: you'll have to walk yourself.)

Love

Dad

PS My bald spot is getting bigger and I can feel the wind on my head when I go out in even the gentlest breeze. Your mother has suggested I set it in place in the mirror in the morning and then spray it solid with hairspray. I think that will look like I am wearing a helmet. Adam says I should get a hat but we do not think we can get one to fit my Hulk-sized head in the shops (when I was in Air Cadets as a teenager, I had to wear a beret cut at the back to fit onto my head). There is some stuff you can get that makes it grow back. I am investigating.

We viewed Michael and Niamh's various moves with some puzzlement. Their time in the cottage in a village just outside Ipswich had been stressful, with cold and damp issues, a difficult landlord and a lost deposit. Bad luck, we thought.

They moved to central Ipswich, supposedly so Michael could be in the thick of things. The move had been a downward one, though, to the cheapest place they could find. It did not work out there either. Living amid a cacophony of throbbing music and sudden shrieks and screams had set Michael's nerves further on edge and they moved on to the maisonette by Ipswich railway station. They had later planned to share a home with a member of Niamh's family in 2012, had given notice and then, for whatever reason, that move had not gone ahead.

By now, there seemed to have been one mess after another. Why not just find a place, settle down and relax there? Why not do something simple for once? Of course, the whole thing was symptomatic of more serious, underlying issues. Michael was still twisting and turning to find some sort of peace. As he could not find it within, he was unlikely to discover it elsewhere.

Money was a core issue too: each place was cheaper, a step down the ladder. I well remember the years when Tracey and I were unemployed, for all of 1983 and 1984, searching the back of the sofa for loose change the day before the benefit cheque arrived, followed by the sharing of carefully weighed and priced baking potatoes from the local greengrocer for an evening meal. This, give or take, was what Michael and Niamh's life must have been like at this time (albeit without the food in Michael's case).

Pride was another issue. They did not want any more help from us, although we stepped forward and offered it (with varying degrees of enthusiasm). The moves to central Ipswich and the railway station were done without our knowledge or help – 'Here's our new address from Friday.' We never visited them at the high-rise and only latterly at the maisonette as tensions eased. Niamh wanted them to stand on their own two feet.

May 2012

Dear Michael,

I just wanted to drop you a line to pick up on one or two things your mother has been mentioning lately (I seem to be out-of-the-loop as I probably wasn't concentrating) . . .

This master's degree – are you up to going to Norwich and back twice a week for two years? That is good to hear and we are happy to pay half of it. What exactly is it? I assume it's not just a repeat and is more specialised? There seems to be confusion as to whether you are doing cartoons or actual film-making – is it *Wallace and Gromit*? I hope it will actually be of some use and will get you a job rather than just being two more years of avoiding work (I am not being rude but you will be nearly twenty-seven by the time it is done). Let me know?

A job from September is good: work, money, food on table, me not paying for everything – excellent. Hopefully, Niamh will like it there. The main thing really is that you are moving forward, some money is coming in and you are getting things together. (I hesitate to say 'at last' but only for a second or two.) All you now need to do is start eating and everyone is happy. (That and a job.)

Love

Dad

x

PS Adam says my bald spot will keep me warm in the summer as it will act as a sort of solar panel. I suggested that was not very funny and that anything he had to say should be constructive. He suggested I cut off bits of 'live' hair and superglued them to the bald patch. I have been giving this some thought. If you think about it, it's not as daft as it first sounds.

This has not been an easy story to tell. It does not unfold in a straight, ever-downwards line. It ebbs and flows: moments of quiet despair mix with sudden hope, irritation turns into humour and often back into anger just as quickly. There were times when everything appeared promising, if not normal.

Close to two years after finishing his degree, Michael had said he wanted to do a master's in animation back up in Norwich. Despite earlier reservations, we were now generally encouraging: it would get him out of the house, give some structure to his week, and start him moving forward again.

Niamh had secured a job from September, which meant that they would, emergencies aside, be self-financing by the autumn of 2012. They moved to another house, slightly nicer, up near a park in Ipswich, and, although we weren't asked to assist with the move, we did visit them there early on. We thought it was a good choice and that they could settle there for a while.

But those moments of hope, our belief that things were improving, were misguided. We allowed ourselves to be deceived. Michael was only ever moving one way and at much the same speed – so slowly that we didn't notice the minute changes. He was steadily losing weight and fading away. Niamh, talking later about this time, said, 'Michael was the thinnest person I'd ever seen.'

Mentally, he was not with us any more. Earlier Father's Days had been spent with get-togethers, meals and presents. This time round, we didn't see him at home for a meal, nothing. There was a present, I was told, but I'd have to go over there to get it. By coincidence, Tracey, Adam and I had gone to a *Doctor Who* show, *The*

Crash of the Elysium, just down the road from them the night before. I had hoped Michael might show up with his present. He didn't, and I couldn't bear to go to his house to fetch it.

22 July 2012

Hello Michael,

A 'just in case' note and checklist as we are away for the next four weekends. We fly out Saturday, via Charlotte, and arrive back on Sunday, 19 August; we land about 8 a.m. and should arrive home at about midday, assuming we do not pull over for a sleep at Clacketts. It depends if I sleep much on the flight – I have not looked to see if the seats are in threes; I assume so, which means I will have to sleep next to a stranger who will no doubt shove his huge fat backside up against my thigh as per last time (cue shudder).

Bernard is going to Barbara and Dawson up at the airbase – he should be fine: Barbara is no-nonsense Yorkshire and he is a big softie. They let Bernard sleep on their bed (when he gets there, he makes a beeline for it). I have given them your number just in case of emergency; I assume Niamh could sort something out with a relative if need be.

Nikki is looking after the house – there is the key in the usual place if you need to come over for any reason. I have hidden a debit card under a cloth at the bottom of the tool box (Jacobs Cream Crackers). You can come get it if need be; the money will be transferred as usual whilst we are away but the bank is so hopeless that I'd rather have a fall-back for you here if anything goes wrong; I do not want to try to do a bank transfer from America.

Did you know Megan has had a baby? Sophie got her something or other for him – Kyle or some other name – and your mother did too. Heavens above, we were just trying to be nice and she turns up with him. Cue embarrassment all round, including Bernard licking the baby's face. She did not stay long – I think he needed feeding or changing – and I do not think we will see her again. It's strange: at one point it felt as though she were family but now it was if someone from your mother's work had come round and we were obliged to be polite to them.

Anyway, if you need to contact us whilst we are over there – point of death only, please – Sophie will have her mobile so go with that. Your mother intends to take hers too but as she cannot work it properly here – she snaps herself when photographing views and we then have to tell her she doesn't really look that bad – there is little chance of her getting it to work there. Last time we went, I 'accidentally' left it in the side of the car at the airport and your mother barely spoke to me for the next twenty-four hours. (That's what's called a 'win-win'.)

All for now. Hope all is well with you and that you are getting yourselves together for what will be a life-changing autumn. I think if you can maybe sort yourself out eating-ise then we can all look forward with some optimism.*

Love

Dad

x

PS *I do not want to be a grandfather yet so please 'hold fire' on that side of things for the time being.

After the strains and tensions of the last two years we wanted to believe Michael's plans would lead to better health, so we tried to keep things breezy, as if all were well.

Maybe living in a new place, with Niamh in a proper job and Michael returning to education with a course he enjoyed, would mean he could get things back on track. 'He just needs a bit more time, that's all.'

We were kidding ourselves. How could we ignore the evidence of our own eyes whenever we saw him? He was beyond thin from top to toe. His head, stripped of flesh, was like a skull.

Out and about, I would see skulls in toy shops, on film posters, and would point and say, 'Michael', hiding terrible thoughts behind awful jokes. As often as not, his name would choke in my throat before it came out.

Michael's body was just skin and bone. His legs were so thin that we couldn't believe they could support him without snapping. I found it hard to look at him and couldn't meet those wounded, defensive eyes. We have photos of him as he declined. I can live with the thinness. It's the eyes that kill me.

No, we didn't believe, not really. We encouraged each other to believe. And we kept on hoping. But we did not really know what would happen. Inside, without saying it to each other, I think we both feared the worst.

So how, seeing this, as parents, could we just stand back, watch and wait? Why did we not rush forward and hug him? Why did we not go to the police or social services and have him taken forcibly to hospital?

My heart beats for my wife and children. Tracey is a warm and loving mother. Sophie and Adam are a good sister and brother. We want only the best for each other. Yet we stood back. I can talk about damaged childhoods and how we shied away from difficult emotional moments. I can tell you that we didn't know what to do for the best and feared we might make things worse. I can stress that we hoped with all our hearts that things would come good. I can give so many reasons.

But the answer to the question 'Why did we not do something, anything?' is a simple one that torments me to this day: 'I don't know.' It's easy, looking back, or from the outside with little knowledge of mental illness and human frailties, to think, We should have said this, and we should have done that. But we didn't. We did what we thought was right at the time. We got it wrong.

August 2012

Dear Michael and Niamh,

A little note – plus a littler enclosure – from us to congratulate you on your engagement. Quite a surprise!

It's all onwards and upwards for you from now on. We hope that Niamh's job will be a happy one and that your master's degree over the next couple of years will lead to you getting the type of film animation work that you want to do.

We all send our love and best wishes and hope that we will see you again soon.

Love

Dad

PS Onwards and upwards!

Tracey, Sophie, Adam, Paul and I came back from Orlando on a Sunday late in August and, an hour or so after our return, Michael and Niamh arrived to tell us their news.

They'd got engaged. They were going to marry somewhere hot and sunny the following summer.

There were smiles and hugs – an arm's length pat on the shoulder from me – laughs and jokes.

I tried to work out what this little lot was going to cost me.

Maybe we didn't believe Michael was on the mend, but Niamh must have done, surely, to have got engaged. She must have known things were on the right track. We hoped that was the case but had doubts.

Did she know something we didn't? Was this a last-ditch attempt to save Michael and turn him around once and for all?

Tracey and I looked at each other.

We turned away.

We smiled at Michael and Niamh and congratulated them.

2 September 2012

Dear Michael,

Day out at Aldeburgh and Thorpeness – have you heard what happened already? I imagine it's all over Sophie's Facebook and what have you. If not, see enclosed photo of me at – in! – Thorpeness Meare, which says it all really.

We parked up by the old Aldeburgh cinema – where we saw that magician? – and worked our way as usual from the bookshop to the knick-knack shop at the top and back down to the upstairs fish and chip shop. Haddock, chips and steamed puddings all round. A quick walk dodging the dog mess on the beach and off we went to Thorpeness.

Arrived, parked easily and we did the usual House in the Clouds and the windmill route march. (Adam and Sophie lagging behind at this point as jam roly-poly and custard start to lie heavy.) Back to Thorpeness Meare and Adam spots the rowing boats. 'Can we?' Your dear mother drops

out, pleading a bad ankle (?) and takes her place at the café
by the meare, a pot of tea for one being brought to the
table.

So me, Sophie and Adam get in the boat, *Dorothy* – ironic
really, given that it ended up somewhere over the rainbow
never to be seen again. Bit of a struggle, with the boat
wobbling all over the place as the three of us climbed in and
got into position. The Saturday lad – about twelve and
seven stone – did his best to steady it for us. Off we went.

It started well enough as we headed off with me pretending to splash them with the oars and the usual cries of 'Oh,
Dad!' We circled the little island with the broken-down
house on it. When it's just me and Adam, Adam gets off and
I row round whilst he crosses to the other side and gets
back in. With three of us wedged solid in position, we
played safe and rowed round together.

Twenty minutes left, we decided to 'explore' one of the
quieter water lanes off to the side. No one about so we
could go at our own speed and take our time. So, there we
were, middle of nowhere, no one in sight, as quiet as you
could imagine, just us, *Dorothy*, the water, and reeds up to
either side shielding us in a little cocoon world.

Sophie then decides she wants to change ends with Adam
– her backside being wedged in the pointy end, Adam in
comparative luxury at the wider end. So they both stand up
– in retrospect, what were we thinking? – and she goes to
shuffle by me. 'Do not wobble the boat, Dad!' (As if.) As she

passes, the boat tilts to one side, steadies in between right-
ing itself and turning over (time passes slowly, I have time
to think, Surely not?) and then it tips over.

It all seems to happen in slow motion. Sophie goes full
length into and under the water. I see the water coming up
to my head – black and surprisingly warm – as it engulfs
my face. Adam somehow manages to avoid going under,
standing up to his waist in the thick black gloop. I get up
and try to stop the boat sinking, heaving at it to keep one
end up and in sight.

So we stand there, now all up to our waists, Sophie and
me with blackened faces. Sophie is covered with indeterminate flora and fauna, bits of it moving slowly across her
forehead (I do not say). Surprisingly, as I would have
expected Sophie to go into meltdown, we all laugh and pose
for Adam's camera photos (see enclosed). Sophie then
phones (phone and camera miraculously intact) your
mother in a panic, asking 'them' (whoever they might be) to
send help. Your mother responds by asking if we need
'Thunderbirds Air Sea Rescue'.

Sophie decides we should call others for help by shouting
'Help' at the top of our voices – clearly, not the best idea as
it would (a) attract attention, (b) give whoever sees us the
best laugh they've had in ages, and (c) not make any difference as no one is going to let us get into their boat and tip
that one over too. I suggested we should just cut our losses
dignity-wise and all swim back, breast stroke, three across,

as it would at least make your mother laugh to see us coming in that way.

Anyway, we decided to climb up onto the bank through the reeds – quite some effort to actually climb out of the water and get up a four-foot bank at right angles; lots of slipping and sliding (Sophie), etc. We did look a sight – Sophie, wet and bedraggled and mascara running all over her face. Was it mascara or goo from the meare? Or some sort of living matter? I did not ask. We made our way back, Sophie phoning and telling your mother to meet us at the car so we could circumnavigate the café where everyone would see us.

Of course, the final humiliation was that the only way we could get back was by walking through the café area, which, inevitably, was near full. We did it with as much dripping dignity as we could muster, strolling through as if it were a perfectly normal end to a day out for us. I then had to go past the boat hut and explain to the man there what had happened. He reacted as though it was an every-day occurrence, asked us where the boat was and sent two teenage lads with what looked like soup ladles to retrieve it. I did not have the heart to say that by now it would have sunk without trace.

So that was our day out as a pre-birthday treat. Adam asked if we could go there again and take another boat out. I suggested we should leave it for a while. Sophie was first to the bathroom when we got back; me and Adam followed

– your dear mother then got the scourer out to clean it.
Happy days!
Love
Dad
x

PS My birthday. Can we resume the traditional celebratory
meal? We can do a Chinese at the house. Let your dear
mother know asap, please. Or just turn up and surprise us
all at seven thirty.

I don't see this story as a misery memoir because at heart we have
always been a happy family and there are many warm memories
from over the years, some coming from our good humour and
cheerfulness in the face of apparent calamity. And there have been
plenty.

On holiday in Knaresborough – someone has to – I had
pretended to jump off the castle walls to my death (always good for
a laugh, that one). In doing so, I had broken my ankle, crying out
as I pulled down my sock to see if the expected bone was protrud-
ing ('Take no notice of Dad, he's just joking'). Four days in hospital, three out and about on crutches, up and down hills, provided
plenty of amusing incidents for the family (though not necessarily
any for me).

Another visit to Yorkshire, on a trip to Haworth, famous, of
course, for the 'Brontë Balti House' (Emily loved a nice *saag*

paneer), our car had been broken into and the thieves had pulled out wires galore in an attempt to start it without success. We spent the rest of the holiday hot-wiring the car ourselves through the Dales. We'd have been even happier if we'd all had baseball caps we could wear back-to-front but you can't have everything.

Yorkshire again – the place is jinxed for us – and Adam ate rat poison that had been left by the holiday home owners for the winter. (I should add the bungalow was not a complete dive but by a river that tended to flood. When it did, the local wildlife headed for the nearest bricks and mortar.) I spent the evening, rather than watching a DVD over a Chinese takeaway, driving frantically round and round York's one-way system searching for the elusive hospital before my youngest son slipped into unconsciousness (not always an easy moment to spot with Adam). It transpired some time later that Adam had not eaten the poison after all but would now quite like a McDonald's.

This latest drama, the Thorpeness sinking, was just another in a long line of things-that-went-wrong, which, one way or the other, went on to become the stuff of family legend. Good times, and long may they continue. How we laughed in the face of disaster.

October 2012

I remember every moment of the day you were born –
when I got home, I wrote it all down so I would never forget
any detail.

I never thought I would do the same the day you died.

I cannot bear the idea of you there in hospital and me here helpless to save you. Waiting for the next text from Niamh.

I've imagined this moment – this year, you always looked thinner, more detached, more vague. I ignored it all. Everything. Just made jokes all the time. I pretended all was well. Hoped it would be.

I thought I would be angry with you. Breaking Mum's heart. I cannot protect her. For casting shadows over Sophie and Adam and the rest of their lives.

I won't let you break my heart. I won't cry for you and I won't tell you I am sorry and I won't tell you I love you either – because of everything you have done to all of us.

I wish I could die for you.

The moment of truth.

Michael had succumbed to pneumonia and was rushed as an emergency to Ipswich Hospital, with a collapsed lung, a failing immune system and a body ready to close down on him.

I texted Niamh: *Is it terminal?*

No.

The truth or a kindness?

I have spent years using notes and letters and checklists, almost obsessively at times, as ways of rationalising and working out my thoughts and feelings and what I should say and do. It's easier than face-to-face talking and hugging, that's for sure. It's what I did again that night as we waited. Words I would never send. Things I would never say. The truth of how I felt though. Written for myself and no one else.

Michael lived.

We did not see him that night but a day or two later when we met in the hospital coffee shop. I struggled to keep my composure at the sight of Niamh pushing him in a wheelchair, our stick-thin, broken boy. I fussed over coffee and biscuits and sugars to distract myself from the horror of it all. There were no jokes that day, but there was an underlying sense of utter relief that, at long last, Michael was where he needed to be to get better.

He had danced with the devil and it had been a long and painful jig. He was told by doctors he might die. He certainly came close. The hospital referred him to the Priory at Chelmsford in Essex. When push came to shove, the NHS saved him.

11 November 2012

Achtung Dummkopf,

Greetings to you in Stalag Priory – I am not sure if this letter will get to you. We pushed it under the barbed wire fence after lights out but I suspect the camp guards will have got to it before the prisoners, and the commandant will have drawn thick black lines through anything relating to escape plans. So, if anything below does not make sense, it is because my references to homemade pickaxes and tunnels and the next full moon have been crossed out.

Good to hear you are alive – we thought you had bailed out. Fini. Kaput. Napoo. Stiff's paddock. Pushing up daisies. A close shave for you, I think. Still, being on the stick-thin side will stand you in good stead when you are ready to escape. Do you even need to dig your way out? You could simply slip through the bars of your cell. When the spot-light turns on you as you break out, you can stand up straight and they will think you are a crack in the wall. Then just turn on your side and you will disappear. Simple.

What do they have you doing? I suppose if you've gone over the top and copped a packet, you'll be on short rations all day. What's the scoff like? Hard tack and skilly? Eat up or else you'll be on jankers. Stick with it and you'll get your soup ticket soon.

Ma, Bunty, Little Willie and the dog say hello and are all well; although the dog's a little ruff. We are hoping to form a blackhand gang to come over to you next Sunday; the day the balloon goes up (your mother's birthday). We'll meet you zero hours six o'clock at the spudhole? We hope you are back in dear old Blighty by Christmas or at least get a chitty for the day.

Compree? Me neither.

Pop

PS Please get better. We love you.

I believe now that, in many cases, there is no rhyme or reason for mental illness. Terrible things happen to people, often as children, and they may be scarred for life, damaged for ever. Equally, awful things happen and others seem to cope somehow, emerging defiant and strong. Life can be good – a loving family, a comfortable home – and depression or whatever strikes regardless. A tiny part of the brain just suddenly clicks the wrong way.

And it is not always something that is easy to identify. The sufferer may not know what is happening to them, and when they eventually do, they may not want those around them, parents, brothers and sisters, close friends, to realise it. Things are kept secret, lies are told, a façade of normality is created and on it goes.

It's often impossible to know what your children are thinking and feeling anyway; some, no doubt, are as happy as the front they present, that they want you to see. Happy, fulfilled, content. Others may be in despair, drinking or taking drugs in secret, behind closed doors. As parents, you want to see the best in your children. So you look for things, perhaps without thinking, that support that.

The fact they may be duping you, even if only to protect you from what is going on, is a terrible thought and it is shocking when you discover it to be the case. Often, that can create anger and ill-feeling at a time when love is needed most.

I also think that before anyone with any form of illness – depression, alcoholism, whatever – can get better, they have to want to do it themselves. You can shout and curse at them. You can beg and plead. You can threaten and punish. Hold them close, walk away, watch and wait and hope as we did: it makes, in my humble view, no real difference. The desire has to come deep from within, not always easy when they may have spent years denying there is any problem at all.

I believe too (and the sermon endeth in a moment) that, as often as not, sufferers need to hit rock bottom before they can turn things around, the point where there is no real alternative but to get better or die. Michael was now at that stage in his journey. Live or die: it was a straight choice for him. It was one that only he could make.

18 November 2012

Dear Michael,

How's life?

Niamh tells your dear mother that we cannot really see you for a little while.

With Sophie now out of halls and into a house of ill repute with various scoundrels and ne'er-do-wells (Olivia, Emily, Lauren, etc.), we've started sending regular food parcels to Durham (it saves her standing in line at the soup kitchens when the shift is over). It's just a mix of treats that she can't really afford on her student loan and the meagre allowance she gets from us. Bread, milk, Jack Daniel's, that sort of thing.

Is there anything you need? We are happy to put something together if you let Niamh know when she next visits and she can relay the list to your dear mother. We can then run it down and leave it with the guards on the gate or Niamh can do the honours. Pads? Pens? Books? Magazines? Cream cakes and cheesy Wotsits?

Ipswich are just rubbish. We still have season tickets but they'd try the patience of a saint. At least Jewell has gone. He had about five right backs at one point. McCarthy will sort it out given time; he plays them in the right places which helps. Maybe, when you are out on bail, you can come along to a match if you like?

So what do you do all day? Niamh seems to think it's quite a strict regime. I suppose they take your belt off you and your shoelaces and don't let you have anything sharp. Is it like McDonald's where everything is plastic and you are trying to cut into a burger with a bendy spoon? Do you get sessions with a trick cyclist to sort out what's what? It's good you have your own room and a telly.

We are all well. Sophie has come down for the weekend. We had a Sunday roast over at the Coach & Horses (Melton), which was nice. We did invite Niamh; hope she said. The pub always seems busy but they can usually fit us in okay. Sophie is going back on the train tomorrow; it works out about the same money-wise as paying for petrol for the car but it's less hassle. If you pay way in advance, it works out at less than half price. Of course, we never do.

I think that's everything. Take care of yourself and hang on in there – it will all come good in the end, I am sure. Let us know what you need.

Love

Dad

x

Although Tracey and I were relieved that Michael was now in the right place, in a structured and closely monitored environment, we realised it could not be easy for him. It was a tough regime at the Priory, with what seemed like every minute of every day being supervised, no lazing about in bed staring at the wall. They got him up early each morning to medicate and weigh him. There were closely supervised mealtimes, as you'd imagine. There was also a mix of activities from yoga and meditation through to group get-togethers where anorexics, alcoholics, drug addicts *et al* would sit in a circle and talk through their anxieties. (Think *One Flew Over the Cuckoo's Nest.*) Our shy and retiring son must have died over and over again from shame and embarrassment.

The highlight of his day was, without doubt, the arrival of Niamh in the evening. By now working – often a 7 a.m. to 7 p.m. job, one way or the other – she visited every day, driving her battered old car down the A12 through rain, sleet and snow flurries on a ninety-mile round trip, night after night.

We were often frustrated that we couldn't see Michael in those early days; we didn't want to push our way in between him and

Niamh in case it caused ill-feeling. But despite our (misguided) negativity towards her, we now started to see her love for him. Love shows itself in many ways, and anyone who has driven up and down that never-ending, bleak and soul-destroying A12 in winter will recognise that this was love of epic proportions. We don't doubt now that it kept Michael going through the darkest of times.

25 November 2012

Dear Michael,

Chin up!

Niamh mentioned you were having something of a tough time. Two weeks? Who told you that? They are doing you no favours. There is no point in going nuts about it (more nuts) as that sort of whirling dervish stuff never helps. You don't want the strait-jacket and hosepipe treatment.

I think you have to try to be realistic. I am sure things will come good for you if you stick at it but you have been a troubled soul, with the benefit of hindsight, going back to at least 2007. We have been sorting old photos we have accumulated over the years and have been filing some photos from the Orlando 'Holiday from Hell' trip with the Robertsons. You were looking quite thin then although we never really noticed.

2007, 8, 9, 10, 11 and 12. You went from being a big healthy lad into a wheelchair, one foot in the grave, less than one month ago. That you got out of Ipswich Hospital alive is an achievement and in such a short time – we had you down and out at Hallowe'en. Twelve-inch needles. Drips. It's a wonder you're here at all. You've done really well.

You know Lily, Sophie's pal? She went into the London Priory a few years back with much the same as you. (Even now she's all ribs and elbows.) She was in for four months. I am sure you will get out before that but you must not expect instant results. Stick with it. Set little targets for yourself.

Is there a TV series you like? We could maybe get you a DVD or two, and when you have had a good day, you could watch an episode. If you have a bad day, you could watch *Downton Abbey*, which is your mother's favourite. You know sometimes you read about someone who has been in a coma for years and they can see and hear everything but are powerless to speak or respond in any way? Watching *Downton Abbey* with your mother is a bit like that.

Talking of your dear mother, I am sure that, if Niamh smuggled it by the guards, you have already opened the 'attached' goodies bag (although new pants and socks do not usually fit into that category). Adam has put in a little note too, I think, and Sophie is sending you something from Durham. What else do you need? Happy to oblige. I assume all Niamh's money is going on daily visits to you; a 100-mile round trip a day must add up.

It would be good to see you soon. Maybe there is an evening or weekend when Niamh does not come down that we could slip in by the guards? Have a talk with Niamh and then she and your dear mother can liaise.

Love

Dad

x

PS I am still swimming weekdays (for all the good it seems to do me weight-wise). There's a sleazy old geezer who goes to the Over 50s Swim on Thursday mornings. Think Benny Hill but without the charm. As this nice-looking woman swam up to him, he said, standing at the shallow end posing hideously in too-tight trunks, 'Darling, where have you been all my life?'

'Hiding.'

Brilliant.

Michael was, strictly speaking, at the Priory on a voluntary basis. When he was in Ipswich Hospital recovering, he was invited to go and stay there. I suspect that, like national service in the 1950s, words such as 'voluntary' and 'invitation' have a range of interpretations at certain times. Had he declined, I do not doubt that I, his next of kin, would have been asked to sign papers to have him taken there by force. I would have done it.

He thought, for some reason, that he was only going to be in for about two weeks – I imagine something like that would have been said to encourage him to agree to go there in the first place. When he realised he was going to be in indefinitely, he flew into a rage leaving his room like the aftermath of a pop star's visit (I am not talking Daniel O'Donnell spilling a cup of tea).

We viewed this, reprobates that we are, with a degree of amusement – the thought of Michael, our mild-mannered son, flying into a fists-of-fury rage was completely at odds with how we saw him. The moment soon passed and was not spoken of again. We should have realised that the incident revealed that Michael didn't really want to be there, getting better, but to get out as soon as he could.

2 December 2012

Dear Michael,

Your dear mother and I met thirty-three years ago this very day (it was a Sunday night too, funnily enough) and we have celebrated today with a breakfast at the Alex, a walk in Rendlesham Forest with Bernard and Adam and will have an Indian takeaway later this evening with a DVD.

Your mother's got us watching *The Tudors* (Henry VIII). Have you seen it? We have had several goes at it over the past year or so. I have seen the first few episodes so many times now I can almost shout out the lines. I also shout out, 'Don't marry him!' at key points but that's to annoy your mother rather than being in the script. We are currently midway through what I think is the third series although, to be honest, I lost track (and the will to live) some time ago.

Do you remember how mad Adam was (I should stop that sentence right there) about Thomas the Tank Engine? I do not know how many little trains he got from that newsagent's up the town. I took him to the pier amusements one Saturday and he got in a terrible temper about something or other – we may have run out of 2ps – and threw his just-bought train into the sea. I could not find it. I ended up looking up the tide times and going back later that afternoon. Incredibly, I found it sticking out of the sand in almost the same place, but it looked about twenty years old. All battered and beaten-up (it's how I feel these days).

Then there was that time you, me, Sophie and Adam went to that Thomas the Tank Engine day at the restored railway place in Essex. (Where was your dear mother: a tennis tournament?) Remember? We had photos taken with the Fat Controller (I was fatter) and I tripped a small girl up (she reminded me of Bonnie Langford) and then Adam weed all over the floor in that train carriage as he spotted the Thomas train going the other way and I had to take my socks off to mop it all up. Happy times!

We are looking forward to seeing you at last. If there is anything you want us to bring (cutting or digging equipment down my trouser legs, etc.), let Niamh know and she can pass the message on. Unlike myself, who has a heart of solid stone, your mother is quite likely to be emotional given half the chance so for goodness' sake try not to say or do anything that might trigger her off or else we are all done for. Try not to look too thin or helpless. Please do not adopt your Stephen Hawking pose. Sit up straight. If we can keep it all brisk and practical, all the better. We won't stop too long just in case.

Hopefully, Sophie can come and see you when she is back in a week or two. The halfwit is usually only a few steps behind her at any given time when she is here so he will no doubt turn up on your doorstep as well. We get no respite, he's here all the time she is and it's driving us mad; your mother thinks I will crack first but I am staying calm to annoy her more (small pleasures).

Enough of this jollity. If you can do some sort of Christmas list that would be helpful. If Niamh is struggling cash-wise, what with all these round trips, let me know on the QT and I will drop you some cashola to give to her under some guise or other. Niamh says to get to you at about seven as you have some sort of communal evening meal with the other inmates at six. What a glorious feast that must be. See you soon.

Love

Dad

PS 2 December is also a sad day as it's the day Uncle Roger died of meningitis. He looked like a young Michael Caine. I think of him sometimes (Roger not Michael Caine). He was only twenty. My earliest memories are all of him: pulling faces at me through Nan's serving hatch, doing magic tricks and playing electric guitar (not all at the same time, of course).

If this were a novel, I would cast myself, old and haggard though I am, as the leading man, the hero. Tall and strong, forever brave and fearless, mild and gentle with small children and kittens. (I would also have flinty blue eyes and a firm jawline, rather than these sagging cheeks, and I would definitely want to have a proper neck, my fat head currently sort of sinking straight into my chest and shoulders.)

In this particular story, I would have spotted what was going wrong for Michael early on, swept in and saved the day; had I done so, the novel would have been a novella wrapped up about three years earlier.

The fact is that I didn't sweep in because I'm not a hero and could never be considered the leading man. I have always found it hard to engage and have wanted to keep emotional and difficult things at arm's length.

Me and my heart of solid stone.

What happened to Michael was, in many ways, not our fault, we did not trigger his downfall. It was something that happened and, even today, Michael doesn't fully understand why. Maybe we could have done more during his descent but Michael didn't want to share his troubles. We didn't want to see them. It sort of unfolded slowly, behind closed doors. Out in the open, we all tried to look the other way.

Now, confronted with seeing him in the Priory, face to face, we were going to have to deal with the reality of what had happened. I had no problem driving there, steely-jawed (ish). I could stride confidently through the car park. I could exude bonhomie with the staff at the door (a warm, velvety laugh). But when I saw Michael, I knew I would struggle not to give myself away and cry.

Heroes, of course, don't cry.

Do they?

9 December 2012

Dear Michael

It was good to see you. I must apologise for my slight wobble on arrival – I was okay coming in (although it was like breaking into Area 51) and the walk through Reception (without wishing to be rude, Night Of The Living Dead) but seeing you sitting up in bed set me off somewhat. At least none of the guards or fellow inmates saw me.

You are in the right place, although it is a bit Stalag Luft, isn't it? We had to speak through some speaker thing several times before being let in and they then checked our bags for contraband and hooch. They even checked us on the way out – I am not sure what they were expecting us to steal: sachets of Complan for Christmas I imagine.

God help me, I must be a stupid man. After all this time, I had not realised you were 'anorexic' as such. We have never thought of the word, let alone used it, even between ourselves. You were 'thin' and 'not eating enough' but never anorexic. How stupid is that? How blind are we? It was only when the woman who brought us through and used the word in conversation that it hit home. (It may have been that which set me off.) That and the other patients who were sitting around the receptionist; you look 'thin' but some of these poor wretches are so weak and sickly that it breaks my heart to see them. Thank goodness you are in there now whilst you have some strength left.

If you are not sure exactly what's going on and how long you will be there for, I can have a word with someone if you like? You mentioned this Dr Webber/Webster? I can drop him an email if you want this week to ask how things are going and what have you? If you speak to him when you next see him and say it's okay to talk to me, I will email him later in the week and report back.

I am sure you can turn this around. If you have had the willpower to eat so little so that you can go from, what, twelve or thirteen stone to, I am guessing, six stone – less? – then you must have the inner strength to turn it back round again. I can barely control what I eat each day let alone day in and day out for five years. I am sure it will take time so do try to do as the doctor says. You just have to focus.

Try not to be distracted by those around you. I am not sure mixing with your fellow inmates is a good idea. Are they a good influence? Clearly, they are all bonkers (political correctness to one side for a moment). If you have one who stabs herself with anything she can get hold of and another who tries to squeeze her way out every time a window is opened, they are probably not good examples. (And no wonder it's so hot in there.) I was amazed at how different people were – I had expected, and saw, quite a lot of Goth and emo girls in and around but there were some older men too. This is all new to me.

I am not very good at this sort of thing, I'm afraid. I am probably not much help to you although I wish I were. I have all the right emotions running through my head but they do not seem to come out very well. Your mother says I am 'faintly autistic' (charming). I shut myself off as a child to protect myself against the hell around me. I remember my father sending me to a psychiatrist when I was about ten. It was all loaded questions about why I didn't want to spend time with my father. I think that, having brought his teenage girlfriend into the house alongside my mother and then throwing my mother out some time later, it might have had something to do with it. Of course, I could not say that. I just withdrew into my shell.

What I am trying to say is that I am happy to talk to Dr Webber/Webster. I am happy to look up anorexia and what it's all about – I assume there is more to this than just wanting to look thin – and I am happy to pay for any treatment you might need. I can drive to and fro to Chelmsford. I can do anything practical and straightforward you want of me but I cannot weep and wail and do that sort of stuff. So tell Niamh to tell your mother to tell me what you want and need and it will be done (so long as it does not involve hugging).

Love

Dad

x

PS 'Love Dad x'. Everyone seems to put 'Love' these days. *Doctor Who* actors signing autographs at the *Doctor Who* Shop. Christmas cards to your mother from people at work she doesn't even like. Waitresses in Frankie & Bennie who want a big tip. All meaningless words. When I write 'Love' I mean 'Love'; I don't just spray it around willy-nilly.

PPS We have not told Grandma about your troubles and woes – it would have broken Granny's heart to have found out and, I suspect, would do much the same with Grandma. I know I always joke about Grandma having been Hitler's girlfriend but the truth is she is all right really (for a German mother-in-law). Maybe, when you are well and looking yourself again, we can invite her up and you and Niamh can drop by to say hello. That would be nice.

Even now, looking back, it defies belief that we did not think of or use the word 'anorexia' until it was mentioned almost casually, in passing, when we arrived at the Priory for the first time. I do not know how that could be over what was almost five years.

I do not understand it.

I cannot really begin to explain it.

I can only try to rationalise it a little by saying that we had no knowledge of anorexia and would have associated it more with teenage girls than boys (the female–male ratio is somewhere between 5:1 and 3:1 depending on what survey you read – and it's not 'just' teenagers either, it runs through the ages).

I would also have seen anorexia as something that was so extreme, so close to death, so final that it was beyond anything that we could imagine or associate with Michael. There wasn't that much wrong with our son that a bit of 'sorting yourself out' and 'cracking on' couldn't fix.

But now we had to face up to it.

We had to accept that Michael was an anorexic.

This was a time of discovery for us. We learned that anorexia, terrible and life-threatening though it is, is often not the core problem but is a symptom of other deep-rooted issues. It's the sufferer's way of trying to handle those other, underlying issues; feelings of worthlessness, depression and negativity.

Michael was not 'bad' or 'useless', although his feelings of low self-esteem made him think he was. He was depressed. He felt he was failing everyone, especially Niamh. As I've stated, not eating was a way of getting some sort of control and of punishing himself. This maelstrom of emotions, on and on, all kept within, torturing himself, had led him to the Priory to be broken down and put back together again.

We knew now that we had to be supportive, to be there for Michael, to do whatever we could, without instructing or advising or guiding or pushing or pulling. We had to be a gentle presence, not too close, not too distant, not exactly encouraging, but just being there. As ever, much of what we tried to do came out in more practical ways – pants and socks from Tracey, offers of DVDs from me – and visits, when he was ready, from Sophie and Adam, who wanted to see him and knew they had to be gently encouraging too. I might have asked when he'd be ready to do some more work for me, which might have been a joke; it is, after all, my default setting at emotional times.

16 December 2012

Dear Michael

What a fun night Friday was – or should I say Saturday morning? Sophie was due to drive back down from Durham early Friday in the clapped-out-mobile but had a long night with the girls the night before and could not decide whether to come down Friday night or Saturday morning. We said don't drive down the A1 on Friday night. It's dark. It's busy. You will be tired. It's dangerous. Do it Saturday morning when you feel fresh. So she left five o'clock Friday night.

Just gone six, we get a series of texts – she's packed up somewhere and is by the side of the road, having called the RAC. No problem, we thought, they will get her started in half an hour (priority being given to stranded young women on their own) and she can carry on or they can, one way or the other, tow her back – we have the full works (me, your dear mother, you, Sophie and, for some reason, the halfwit seems to be on it too).

Just gone seven, still no sign of their arrival. Sophie seems confused as to where she is – why she could not use the sat-nav thing on her phone we never know (nor did we ever find out, neither of us daring to ask her afterwards for fear she might blow). She thinks it might be Grantham, or somewhere near Peterborough. But it's on a main road (so that narrowed it down quite a lot). Apparently, the RAC had asked her to find a number on some road markings by the side of the road and she had given them those and they were on their way. Not long now.

Eight o'clock, still no sign. I spoke to her and was trying to work out where she could be having driven an hour or so from Durham. I had her somewhere on the A1 near Sheffield; remember those big chimney pot things? Anyhow, I got on the phone and shouted down it at the RAC, who said they had sent someone to Peterborough in error and they were now on the way to her. Panic over.

Eight thirty, me, Adam and your mother are watching a *Hancock* – the one where he is doing a stand-up routine in a Spanish nightclub and no one understands him – and the phone goes. Sophie says the RAC have called and said she had broken down near Stamford and they would be an hour and a half to get to her. I lost my patience at this point and decided I would go and get her myself. I wanted to shout at this point so I did.

Off I went, thinking that Cambridge Services are about an hour and a quarter and, with a bit of luck, the RAC will get to her and get her going and we can meet there for a second dinner (your mother having done some sort of stir-fry thing, small bowl, earlier). They do a nice crumble at Cambridge Services. Lovely with a bit of custard. So, over the Orwell Bridge we go and she calls again. Long story, but apparently she is not in Stamford (100 miles, hour and a half) but in Pontefract (200 miles, three hours). She packed up just after the A1 turn-off for the M62. But the good news is that the RAC are on their way. We'd heard that before so I carried on driving.

I arrived at 12.37 a.m. having, inevitably, got mixed up in the A1-M62 I-want-to-go-that-way-but-the-road-is-taking-me-this-way tangle. The RAC had got there a while before (not much) and told her the radiator was shot to pieces and had towed the car and her to a petrol station forecourt. I was to bring her home and to leave her keys with the lad behind the desk and the RAC would pick them up and bring the car home the next day.

Quite a long journey home – by the end of it, the windows were all open, my arm was out of mine and the CD was on at just about the highest volume; all I needed was a baseball cap and I could have been spending the evening roaring round the McDonald's car park. We got back at 3.40 a.m. Strangely, the halfwit, who usually turns up five minutes after she gets back, did not on this occasion.

And what of you? Will we see you at Christmas? Can we come in or give Niamh presents? It would be good to do something as a family on at least one of the days. I can't say having Christmas lunch in the Priory is high on my bucket list, if at all, but we will give it a go. Let us know asap, please.

Love

Dad

x

PS I have emailed this Dr Webster to ask for an overview but have not yet heard back. Do you want to give him the thumbs-up to reply and we can then get some idea of how things are going and how long you will be in for?

Michael came out of the Priory from Christmas Eve to Boxing Day, which he spent at his home with Niamh. There were some warm and caring text messages between him and Tracey over this time but we did not see him. We wanted to, but we kept away to give him space and time to be with Niamh.

It's been a family tradition, since Michael was small, for me to take the children to see a Christmas film at the cinema on Christmas Eve afternoon (Tracey doing things with turkeys and pies and puddings meanwhile). This was the first time in twenty years that Michael had not been with us and I missed him.

Was this time out a sign that he was close to being better? No. I talked later on the phone at some length with the head honcho at the Priory, who seemed to be walking something of a tightrope with Michael at this time.

Michael had not expected to be in the Priory for long and had reacted badly when he found out he would be in there, most likely, for months. If Michael had not been released at Christmas, on trust that he would go back as promised, it was feared he might walk out altogether.

(I had images of Michael on the run in some sort of *Fugitive*-style movie but the moment soon passed.)

If he did walk out, or did not come back after Christmas, they would have moved quickly to have him sectioned, locked up in the Priory on a committed rather than a voluntary basis; a huge backward step for everyone.

On Boxing Day evening, he climbed into Niamh's ropey old car and she drove him the long journey back to the institution. What a journey – painful, heart-breaking, hopeful, fearful and then some – that must have been for them.

2013

The year began full of promise. Tracey and I did a lot of soul-searching over everything that had happened. Things had gone horribly awry for Michael, yet Sophie seemed to be flourishing and things were going well now for Adam. So was it us as parents, was it Michael or was it that, sometimes, bad stuff just happens for no good reason? We had so few answers.

Some couples might have taken to counselling to work through these issues, but not us. We saw ourselves as strong and capable and able to work things out between ourselves. Sophie and Adam had had the same sort of childhood as Michael and had turned out just fine. Nothing bad had happened to Michael at any time, so far as we knew, and there was no logic at all behind any of it. That was the thing, really: it made no sense. It just happened. It was the way it was.

But Michael was in the right place and his issues were being tackled at last. He was, we thought, comfortable, albeit not that happy, in the Priory and would be there until he was better. He would resume his master's degree when he was fit and well. Niamh was earning and could support them. And they had their life to look forward to. We hoped 2013 would be a good year and, for once, it was.

6 January 2013

Dear Michael,

We are really pleased that you got out over Christmas but it would have been nice for us all to have seen something of you; at least things are going in the right direction at last.

You wanted to know exactly what it was I had said to Dr Webster. Here, word for word, is what I emailed.

Dear Dr Webster,

We are Michael Maitland's parents and wish to make an observation for you to consider. So far as we are aware, Michael was a fit and happy young man up to 2007. He met his fiancée, Niamh, in 2007. In those days, Michael spoke more freely with us and talked of his early relationship with her. At the time, she seemed a normal-sized girl to us but, as with Michael, soon became much thinner. We do wonder whether Niamh may have been the trigger for what has happened since.

Niamh has, in our view, exerted total control over Michael over the past five years and we are not sure that this is beneficial for Michael. This seems to continue up to and including his stay in the Priory. Everything seems to suggest that he needs to get Niamh's agreement to do anything.

It may be that we have misjudged Niamh. Although there have been various matters over the years that have made us feel ill at ease, it may be that, without Niamh, Michael would not even have got this far. Positive or negative, we cannot help but feel Niamh is a key factor in all of this and, as such, would ask you to give this your consideration.

Yours,

Iain and Tracey Maitland

His reply was as follows:

Dear Mr and Mrs Maitland

Thank you for taking the time to put your thoughts in an email. It is always very useful for us to get the opinions of close family members and I want to let you know that I will factor these into how we aim to help Michael.

Thank you once again.

I just wanted to put our concerns over. We have hinted at these over the years. Perhaps more so, there have been occasions when I have asked if you (you alone) wanted to come back home and start over. Clearly, it's been difficult to raise this matter with you to any great degree.

It was written simply to try to add something to Dr Webster's (limited) knowledge (of you) and to assist him in helping you to get better. You should take it in the spirit it was meant. After all, we all want you to get well soon.

Love

Dad

x

PS Are you now going to get regular time out? If so, and it is when Niamh is working, I'd be happy to run down and pick you up and take you back to Ipswich. I can run you back down too if you wish. You only have to ask. It might be nice – like when we used to go to the football in Manchester (although hopefully you can stay awake during the journey and I can avoid running out of petrol).

We thought for a very long time – from the early signs right through to Michael going into the Priory when we felt we could not get near him because Niamh visited every night – that Niamh may well have been behind Michael's downfall. People tend to search for someone to blame for everything, including their own failings.

There were signs: Niamh had become much thinner (so we thought her diet had triggered Michael's), everything had to be approved by Niamh and nothing could be said or done without her say-so.

The reality, as we see now, was quite different, almost the opposite. Michael wanted to keep his troubles between himself and Niamh for as long as he could – and he did, until the point of collapse. He did not want us to know. He did not want us to try to help. He wanted us kept away. All Niamh did was to love him, protect him, shield him, care for him and take charge of everything for him at his request. Hardly a malign influence, just a purely loving one.

If Niamh had not been there, what would have happened to Michael on his own? Would he have turned to us, allowed us to help him if we could, got things sorted more quickly? Would he have stood on his own two feet? I like to think so but, in my heart, I suspect the worst, and that, without Niamh and not wanting to turn to us, Michael might have died somewhere out there on his own.

13 January 2013

Dear Michael,

I hope you are well and that you will be able to start coming out into the daylight soon. I am happy to pick you up and/or drop you off if you are let loose whilst Niamh is working. Meantime, some news for you from us here at Three Mile Island.

Sophie ran down on Friday in the car (went back this
afternoon, we think) to see some friends for a birthday
thing and, as always, the halfwit arrived literally six
minutes after she did just as we were sitting down to eat;
he ended up having half of her food and more besides. I
could tell from your dear mother's face that we were close
to breaking point on this.

He has to all intents and purposes moved in whenever
she is here. He arrives just after her, eats the food, stays
the night and then goes off without saying a word. Your
mother never gets a chance to talk to Sophie on her own
any more. He can even get in the house and up the stairs
without Bernard hearing and Adam has seen him walking crab-like sideways up the staircase so as not to be
heard.

As I have said, he is not an unpleasant fellow: he does not
shout and swear or drink or take drugs or treat her badly
but he is deadly dull – by God, he is dull – and they are not
a good match. She is hard-working, driven, and wants to be
the best that she can be. He is happy to drift along. She will
outgrow him in time and I just hope it is before they are
stuck in the one-bed mid-terrace with two kids, mangy
mutts and an annual holiday on Canvey Island.

We have, for some time, been meaning to try to ease him
out a little so he is not a permanent fixture when she
finishes her degree. If he is *in situ* then, we will never get
him out and it will be that much harder for her to end

things if he is living here when she comes to her senses. Anyway, Sophie seemed to spot your mother was unhappy (sighs, stares, pointed remarks) and there was something of a confrontation at the tennis club tuck shop (your mother and Nikki still run it on Saturday mornings). Your mother indicated he was still welcome here but only three or four nights a week and for occasional meals; Sophie, naturally enough, went nuclear, and we have had shoutings and Lord knows what. Sophie went off shortly thereafter and has not been seen here since.

Quite what will happen next beats me. Hopefully, it will all sort of fall back into place by the time Sophie next comes down in about March. Whether he will reappear straight away or not is another matter. We live in hope.

So, whatever it is like in Stalag Priory, it's been better there than here, that's for sure. Do pass on any messages via Niamh – do you need anything?

Love

Dad

x

PS You are one week closer to getting out than you were last weekend, and when I write again next weekend, you will be two weeks closer than you were just a week ago. It's like time-travelling, isn't it?

Our style of parenting was such that we were laid-back about comings and goings at home over the years. Friends were welcome to stay over, fridges could be raided, meals could be cooked and, as long as someone sometimes walked the dog for me, we were free and easy with all of that. We invited the children's friends for days out, on holidays with us and, by and large, were fairly liberal parents.

Sometimes it would backfire and we would end up living in a madhouse but things were generally good. Despite my dreadful jibes, Paul was a good lad. Yet there was a growing sense that we were being railroaded into having Sophie and Paul living with us in due course. We muttered between ourselves about this and, with me as the 'bad cop' and Tracey the opposite, I think I was expected to blow spectacularly at some point. As it was, it was Tracey. And it was magnificent.

Later, some time later, Sophie and Paul did break up, quite suddenly and, by then, unexpectedly. Tracey and I saw him in Ipswich a week or two after and we smiled and waved at each other from a distance, neither of us being sure of the other's reaction. That same day, he sent a warm and beautiful text to Tracey, and I then emailed him my thanks.

Hi
That was a lovely text to Tracey – thank you for it.
    We were not sure if to stop or not – we will next time.
    I hope you are at least okay-ish – this must be an extremely

difficult time for you. It must be awful to think your life is going in one direction and then discover suddenly it is not.

It seemed to come out of the blue – as far as we knew, you were moving in together from September. We'd offered to match whatever you'd saved and I had been pointing out 'good' and 'bad' houses that were coming up for sale.

We are sorry things went a bit wonky between us – going back a bit, we were trying to ease away from a scenario where you effectively moved in as, if you then broke up after Durham, it would have been that much harder.

As it happens, that seems to have been what happened although we take no pleasure from it. I suspect it is all done and dusted and we are sorry about that. I guess all I can say is that she was always fiercely protective of you at all times, even at the mildest comment.

I think it is good that you are doing exams and things are looking bright for you work-wise. I hope your personal life goes well and that you find happiness. We send you love and best wishes and wish you well for the future.

Iain

We have not seen Paul since but, as with Lee and Henry before him, and although they were not right for our brilliantly bonkers Sophie, we seemed to have formed an attachment to and had a fondness for him. Paul was the nicest of guys.

20 January 2013

Dear Michael,

Niamh says you might be coming out on Friday for the weekend and that I can come and get you at about 10 a.m.? Wee, wee wee! That is just perfect. I can drop Adam at St Jo's, come and have a scoff and a read at the McDonald's at Chelmsford turn-off and get to you for ten. I will wait in the car park (if they don't let you out, shin down the drainpipe and we'll make a run for it, *Thelma and Louise*-style).

Maybe you can have a talk with Dr Webster to get some idea of when you will be fully released and let me know Friday – I assume you will have weekends out for a month or two and then longer periods until they finally let you go completely. You should be out in good time for August, though, I would imagine?

I'm not convinced that this course is really going to lead to a full-time job with Walt Disney or other big-name studio. I do not want to be too downbeat at this time but I do not think you should pin all your hopes and dreams on it. But I think that if you can get back on it again – see if they will let you do the first term again no charge? – then it will give some structure to your week-to-week life. If you can go once or twice a week then that, with what you do for me, should keep you fairly busy and organised. You want to avoid having too much free time. Get on with things rather than thinking too much.

I am not sure if/how to talk to you about all that has happened over the past few years or if we need to; the (not) eating, the reasons behind it, the things that have gone wrong between us and so on. I am afraid I have always been very lacklustre in the whole range of 'embarrassing conversation' type things; birds and the bees, (not) taking drugs and the whole 'women' business. I am probably useless and inadequate as a father when it comes to that side of life. I do not really know if you want to talk about it (with me) anyway, but if you do, I will give it a go (we will need to talk about something on the journey unless you plan to fall asleep straight away as you always used to do). I will leave it to you to broach any subject; if you want to, of course.

See you Friday, 10 a.m.

Love

Dad

xxx

After a while, as he started to cope with his mental issues and to put on a little weight, Michael was allowed out for weekends, with me collecting him on Friday mornings and Niamh taking him back on Sunday evenings.

We started to talk at these times, tentatively at first but with more confidence later. I am not sure that either of us really looked forward to the early conversations as they covered difficult and emotional topics. I remember odd snippets.

'Are you putting on weight?'

'A bit. It goes on the organs first. It'll be a while before it shows.'

'I always thought it was Niamh.'

'No, she always wanted to be friends with everyone.'

'We blamed her.'

'It was all me.'

'Have you made us a wonky pot?'

(Laughs.)'No.'

To be honest, we tended not to look at each other but out of the side windows instead (not the easiest thing to do when you're driving at 70 m.p.h. up the A12).

We did not dwell on the past, the ifs, buts and maybes, and the things we could have said and done that might or might not have prevented this outcome.

But we talked, with words of regret and sorrow hanging there but unspoken, and that, the talking, the chatting, the eventual moving on to more mundane and trivial matters of football, films and things we might do in the future, was what felt important. It was from this point that Tracey's and my relationship with Michael, and Niamh, started to change and improve.

It changed us too, Tracey and me, Sophie and Adam. We are conscious that mental illness – one in four people experience some form of it each year – is part of our daily lives now.

We are more supportive and encouraging. We are more open. I still struggle with face-to-face talks and all of that. But I can shout up the stairs, 'Are you all right?' with the best of them and I am better at engaging one-on-one in small-talk about what we're doing and the films we're going to see together at the weekend.

It is not always easy. We are often trapped within our own emotional shortcomings. There was a time, not so very long ago, when Michael came home to live with us. As he arrived, sitting hunched in the car next to Tracey, his suitcases and belongings stacked in the boot, I came out of the house to greet them. Tracey, getting out of the car first, mouthed to me that I was to hug him. I couldn't bring myself to do it. Tracey managed to coax Michael out of the car, signalling to me again, behind his back: hug him. I busied myself with the bags in the boot. At Tracey's third gesture, with me now on the brink of breaking down, I moved forward and patted him several times on the shoulder, unable to speak. We went into the house. The three children circled each other and hugged.

I do my best. I try to talk to Michael as a normal person who just happens to have a mental illness rather than as a mentally ill person who has to be spoken to 'normally', with carefully picked words in hushed tones.

There are still jokes, of course. How could there not be? However, I do now try to think before I speak. I think that's often for the best.

25 February 2013

Dear Michael

I think, probably, this will be my last letter; when all is said and done, it is better to talk. Here, though, as promised, is the latest/last round of emails I have exchanged with Dr Webster so you know exactly what's what and where we are at.

> Dr Webster,
>
> You were kind enough to email me a month or two ago about Michael. I wanted, if I may, just to check progress with you.
>
> Michael looks a little better and I am now picking him up on Friday mornings and we chat comfortably on the way home. We then see Michael and Niamh for lunch or coffee on Saturday or Sunday and that has helped to rebuild things. He tells us he is progressing well.
>
> So, as far as we can see, there are encouraging signs. Is that the case with you?
>
> Regards
>
> Iain Maitland

This is his reply (and it is a gold star for you):

> Hi Mr Maitland
>
> Thank you for your email; forgive the delay in responding.

I am extremely pleased with Michael's progress and as I'm sure you have noticed his true personality is returning and his dependence on Niamh is abating. She seems somewhat relieved with this and I suspect the anorexia ended up grossly exaggerating any natural dependent features within his usual personality. We are doing a lot of work around this and him eating alone, and in fairness he has been very humble and brave regarding dealing with it.

Thus, all in all, I feel he is doing very well; I am aiming to discharge him soon and what's left of the disorder can be dealt with in the community.

Dr Peter Webster

Lead Consultant Psychiatrist in Eating Disorders

The Priory Hospital Chelmsford

I then wrote:

Hi

Thank you for everything you have done for Michael – although a simple thank you really doesn't do justice to how grateful we are.

Best wishes

Iain and Tracey Maitland

And finally (get that big trumpet out):

Hi Mr Maitland

It's been a real pleasure, particularly to see how his personality has grown and returned to an adult. I am very pleased for you all and hope it all works out OK. If there's a slip-up we are always here.

It must be lovely to have your son back!

All the best

Dr Peter Webster

Lead Consultant Psychiatrist in Eating Disorders

The Priory Hospital Chelmsford

Love

Dad

x

PS See you on Friday, number one son, 10 a.m.

I've thought hard about how to finish our bittersweet story and what I wanted to say and, also, what you might want me to say (bearing in mind I do not do 'the emotional stuff').

Michael is a good person who lives with mental illness. It's a constant test for him, day in, day out.

I am often misguided and wrong but I believe my heart is in the right place.

Tracey, Sophie and Adam: we are a nice family doing our best to be kind and happy.

So how do I end? Back where we started. It's about love, remember. That's all that matters.

(I rather suspect you wanted me to end with some sort of emotional 'I love you' message to Michael but I am not going to. I don't need to. He knows.)

THE PRIORY: MICHAEL MAITLAND,
IN HIS OWN WORDS

While in the Priory I kept a daily diary. I wanted to write about my experiences staying there so that I'm now able to look back at how things have changed since then. Diary writing forms part of the treatment and I would record my thoughts and feelings, my anxieties and observations, and also my frequent impatience to leave as soon as I could.

The Butterfly of Freedom (my diary starts with this poem)

> *Why do you fly outside the box?*
> *I fly outside the box because I can,*
> *But we know the box, we are safe inside the box,*
> *That, my friend, is why I leave it.*
> *For you may be safe, but I am free!*

Arriving at the Priory, I went in with Pepsi and sweets, which they took off me straight away. The first couple of days they literally give you minimal food – I was eating less than I would at home. I remember seeing Niamh walk away outside. She was crying and I was stuck with the other loons.

I felt very lonely and decided to watch the whole Lord of the Rings *trilogy back-to-back in my room. That made me feel better, at least for a bit. Niamh came over in the evening and had made me an Xmas calendar. Niamh coming here is the only thing keeping me going at the moment. Really dreading the thought of having to be here during Xmas.*

It really feels like being in prison. You are checked up on and watched all the time, especially during meals. Snacks are checked, staff come into your bedroom every fifteen minutes, and it's slowly becoming more apparent that I'm going to be here far longer than two weeks.

I pretty much seem to be having injections every single day at the moment, having blood taken.

You are marched through locked corridors in single file to the café area. After each meal we have to sit around in a group for forty-five minutes and talk – most of the time we sit awkwardly.

I met a lovely older lady called Louise, who has had issues for many years. Not sure how old she is, maybe sixty. She seemed very scary but turned out to be one of the kindest people I have ever met. She had eating problems along with other things like agrophobia, the fear of leaving her house and going outside.

It's snowing today and I'm worried about Niamh driving here later.

I weigh 45.7 kilos. Body image session today. We get to see Dr Webster once a week for an update: I want to ask what is happening. This can be very frustrating, seeing him just once a week as time is very slow.

I want to see my family but I feel ashamed and embarrassed for them to see me here. I want my brother and sister to come but they might find it shocking. I am sitting here on my bed and can hear patients screaming and swearing in the distance (alcoholics).

I have a guy called Richard who does CBT (cognitive behavioural therapy) – he is great and helps me a lot. He is probably the best person I have met and has really started to help me feel better about myself. He also runs some of the group sessions here during the day.

I just found out I have to drop out of my master's – I feel ashamed as I'm completely letting everyone down. Niamh assures me it's the best thing and I will be able to go back to it.

Talk with Dr Webster didn't go well to say the least – he told me I'm going to be here until after Xmas.

I got to pop out in the car with Niamh. She took a picture of us and put it on Instagram – I think my parents thought I had made a run for it ha-ha – whereas we just sat in Costa.

Woken at 6 a.m. and stripped down to nothing but my boxers. Today we are getting weighed. You have to stand in front of the nurse in the freezing cold. Then a bit later I join the queue of loons to pick up my medication. Fun times.

I have made a really good friend called Tom. He is older than me and has a beard that is literally about fifty centimetres long. He used to be a taxi driver, but things got so bad for him that he could barely walk upstairs any more.

Niamh gets to come over once a week for dinner – the highlight of my week.

Get to go home for the night – staff make me fill out a form asking if I'm planning on running away – like I would tell you, lol. They also check your bags like you're some sort of criminal.

Got to go with my 'rehab' group to town and look round the shops. I am not good at buying myself stuff so I just look. Our group must look like a right bunch of weirdos walking around.

Sitting at breakfast and we notice Angie is missing. I look outside and see her legging it down the front drive in her dressing gown – members of staff then chase her.

I can now have lunch and tea unsupervised in the restaurant. I was sat with the other loons, like alcoholics and drug-users. One of the drug addicts became increasingly angry before throwing his dinner on the floor. He was shouting at his dinner saying it was cold whilst I sat there quietly looking at the table in front of me.

My time in the Priory certainly wasn't easy and is one of the hardest things I've had to experience in my life. I still think about my time there and always will. To this day, I keep a little red meal token I got there in my pocket to remind me of what I went through and how far I've come.

AFTERWORD

I t's now July 2016, three years on, and we are all still here. I would like to say we've all lived happily ever after but it's not quite true, not yet anyway.

I no longer write health, wealth and happiness articles for newsletters and the like. The internet effectively killed off *Reader's Digest*-type information that can be accessed easily via Google. I now earn a living writing about UK and overseas property and putting developers and investors together.

Tracey is still a teaching assistant at the local primary school. We have now been together for almost thirty-seven years and will, hopefully, like the lovers in *The Notebook*, die together in our eighties.

Sophie spent three years at Durham University. As with Michael, I offered her my own unique brand of guidance and advice on life at times, via the odd letter, emails and the occasional shouting match, all of which she ignored completely. She left with a 2.1 degree, completed a teacher training course, won some awards, and is now a mature and sensible primary school teacher. She has a boyfriend, Glyn, who we think is 'the one'.

Adam did well enough in his GCSEs, better than the Ipswich School dog anyway (we think). He is now doing A levels at a sixth-form college.

He has a girlfriend, Sophie (a.k.a. 'Normal Sophie'), who seems nice; he tries to keep her away from us as much as possible in case I embarrass him with my Penguin impression from the 1960s *Batman* series.

Niamh has moved on and now lives and works abroad. She turned out to be nicer than we thought and almost certainly went to Hell and back many times to save Michael's life. Hers was a loving influence.

And Michael? After leaving the Priory, having spent five months there, Michael got better for a while, putting on a little weight, starting to draw again and resuming his master's degree. Then, as time passed, things took another downturn and, two years later, he went to the edge of grief and sanity. This time, though, we all stepped forward and acted decisively.

We went into the abyss together in the middle of 2015 and thought this was the end of him. Nights of hiding tablets and knives, lying awake at 2 a.m. listening for him, and mornings where we'd talk through desperate thoughts and feelings. Somehow, we just about got things right between us. In 2016, Michael now seems to be in the early stages of recovery again. He completed his master's, and works as an illustrator.

But all of that – the grief, the madness, the abyss, the recovery – is another story for another time. For now, we are alive and well. We laugh. We talk more openly. We eat. We put the rubbish out. We go up the town together. We come home. We get on with things. We are mostly happy. We are together. We are a family.

Iain Maitland
Suffolk, 2016

PS Bernard's here too. And he's still staring at me.

IN CONVERSATION WITH MICHAEL MAITLAND

I could not have written a book as intimate and revealing as this without the love and wholehearted support of my family. I have had that from start to finish and could not have wished for any more from them.

I wrote, early on, that this story is seen and told from one side, mine. And, as stated, I may well be an unreliable narrator. Everyone recalls events in different ways, from their own viewpoint. Memory is a strange thing. I think it is human nature to rewrite memories mentally to make ourselves seem cleverer, more successful and more heroic. I have tried to avoid that.

Before showing the final script to the family, I wanted Michael to read it, to give him the chance to correct things and to put his side of the story. His thoughts are revealed in this conversation.

Michael asked me to snip out two sentences. Tracey and Sophie both asked me to remove one line each. Other than those tweaks, the book is as I wanted to present it. My family is happy and at ease with it. Sophie summed it up in a text *We're proud of you*, as I am of them.

Iain: So (*laughs*), who'd have thought? What do you think of it?

Michael: It made me laugh a lot as well as remembering sad times. I found it hard to read in places, but it's probably going to be hardest for me to read out of anybody. It's all obviously from your perspective, which I considered whilst reading it, and there's obviously more that was experienced on my side of things. Overall, I love it and think it has a perfect balance of humour, insight and tragic moments but it still ends on a positive note.

Iain: I've tried to tell the story truthfully as I see it but without 'crossing the line', without being too graphic. Does my perception of what happened sit reasonably well alongside your own reality?

Michael: I tried to read it knowing it's how you see things, rather than my own experiences. I think that, overall, it's a fair account of what has happened.

Iain: Looking at what happened to you, was there a particular trigger or cause for it all?

Michael: For some people there may be something that obviously sticks out but from my experience it just tended to be a culmination of various things. From the people I've met and talked to along the way, who have suffered, you can often never pinpoint one thing, but a possible mix of things, whether it's the people you're around, school, job, lifestyle or how confident you are, I guess.

Iain: Could any of it have been avoided do you think or was this all just meant to be?

Michael: I don't know if it can be avoided. There are probably obvious things such as going to the doctor that people could do

to try and stop what is going to happen, but I think it was probably meant to be.

People with mental illness still get looked at differently, in
my opinion, and it is therefore already hard to reach out for
help. So you are already in a difficult situation. Even if you do
think you may be suffering, you may not find it easy to say
anything.

I know from having depression, it was hard to say anything to
anyone apart from Niamh because she understood, whereas
others may think, Why don't you just get on with it? Or be
happy? This isn't the right thing to do.

Iain: No, I realise now that's pretty much the worst thing that I
used to say to you . . . It took me a while, until the Priory
really . . . What advice could you give to those suffering from
mental illness?

Michael: If you are suffering from mental illness, it feels like it's
impossible to talk to anyone about it. It's important that you at
least try to. Some people won't understand what you're going
through but there are people in the same boat as you.

It's also important to try and not hate yourself. You have to try
and think that you're a worthwhile person who has people who
care about you. Keep trying different methods, talk to people,
until you find something that works for you. It might take a
while, but I think there is something that can work for
everyone.

Iain: Later, in 2015, when we were looking for help somewhat
urgently, it seemed to me that those who had experienced

mental health issues themselves were often better placed to assist than GPs. What are your thoughts on that?

Michael: Yes, I agree with that. I think that doctors can help to some degree and might suggest medication. I have tried many different types of medication and, yes, they can work, but it's not ideal because it's only really a temporary fix. I think it's better to find alternative ways of coping.

I have heard that people feel that things like meditation, yoga and exercise can also help. It's very important to keep looking until you find what's right for you, whether it's a specific activity, or possibly someone to talk to that has knowledge and experience with the issue. Then if you can learn methods you can use to help yourself, you can start to feel more positive on your own.

(*Iain*: For those struggling with mental illness right now, I should say here I've been told that, in the darkest times, sufferers and/or their loved ones can go to their GP and ask to be referred urgently to what's known as the crisis team. I believe it's called the Access and Assessment Team [AAT] in Suffolk and may be known as something similar in other places. They should come out near enough straight away to assess and offer help. GPs should also be able to direct sufferers and loved ones towards support groups, for people with eating disorders, for example. In an emergency, people can also Google 'crisis team' or 'crisis team Suffolk', or whatever part of the country they are in, and that should generate various leads for those seeking urgent help.)

Iain: As for parents, family and friends, what is 'the right thing' to do?

Michael: I would say that if you know someone who is suffering, or you think might be, then don't force anything. Just be there for them, whether that's by asking if they're okay, listening or just being supportive (like giving a hug, not a Maitland thing to do, ha!).

If someone is suffering, it will mean the world to them to know that someone is there, who cares enough to listen but not push. When you reach out to someone suffering it will mean a lot. Times when I have felt awful and, say, Sophie or Adam ask if I want to see a film or something, it makes me feel a lot better because it's nice knowing there is someone there.

Iain: What other things could people try that might help?

Michael: Again, it's hard to pick one particular thing that will help. Everyone suffering with mental issues will find some more useful than others. The main thing I'd recommend is to talk to someone. Whether it's your partner, family, doctor or whoever, it's important to reach out.

I have tried lots of things including doctors, medication, CBT [Cognitive Behavioural Therapy], hypnotherapy and many others. For me, the most helpful has been hypnotherapy for sure. It may take some time exploring different people and places before something clicks. This can be horrible as you may think you're too crazy for anything to work but if you keep trying there will be something.

Iain: Do you still have mental health issues?

Michael: Yes, I do, and I know that I always will, just not to the degree that I have experienced. I have lost a lot from mental illness and have been at rock bottom. I still have struggles but the worst is over, I like to think. Depression is the main thing I know is always there, and it's just a case of trying to stay out of that as much as possible.

Iain: And how do you stay out of that?

Michael: I think it's important to learn to stay as positive as possible and know that you're not alone. I find that staying busy with things, but still recognising your limits, is important. If there's something you enjoy doing, then do it, or at least try to have a go at it.

If I'm feeling rubbish, then I'll go for a walk, see a film or hang out with Adam. I lost interest in loads of things over the time I was depressed, like illustration, films or gaming. Recently, I've really tried to do these things again and it seems to make me feel better. I'm even getting to write for video game websites and create content, which I love.

Also, it's important to remember the past but not dwell on it. I'm so grateful for what Niamh did for me and am so sorry for what happened. I still feel utterly guilty but you have to realise it's not your fault. I feel lonely a lot but I always try to remember that there are people around me that care.

The most important thing, though, and Niamh always tried to tell me this, you have to learn how to like yourself. If you don't like yourself, or take care of yourself then, no matter how much anyone else loves you, you will not feel better. Find some sort of self-worth.

Iain: I guess it just has to come from within, really. You can't force someone to be happy from outside. How do you see the years ahead?

Michael: I don't know for sure. I never thought I would go through what I have or lose everything pretty much. I would like to hopefully do more illustration and create more video game content. I would love to work in the video games entertainment industry (like IGN).

I would also like to get my own place again at some point, as I think it's important for me to have independence and be able to grow. Hopefully I will make some friends, if they are mental enough to like me (lol).

I know that mental illness is something that will always be there. I know that depression will always be there, but I'm much better at managing it. I know that things can only get better. I'm hopeful for the future.

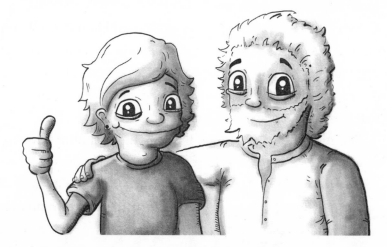

An invitation from the publisher

Join us at www.hodder.co.uk, or follow us
on Twitter @hodderbooks to be a part of
our community of people who love the very
best in books and reading.

Whether you want to discover more about a book
or an author, watch trailers and interviews, have the
chance to win early limited editions, or simply browse
our expert readers' selection of the very best books,
we think you'll find what you're looking for.

And if you don't, that's the place to tell us what's missing.

We love what we do, and we'd love you to be a part of it.

www.hodder.co.uk

 @hodderbooks

HodderBooks

 HodderBooks